ANS GIBSON

How I Defeated Lyme Disease

A holistic journey that turned Lyme from a curse to a blessing

First edition

ISBN: 9780578711607

Editing by Daniel Stokarski

This book was professionally typeset on Reedsy.
Find out more at *reedsy.com*

This book is dedicated to Elizabeth Morrow for your love and support throughout the years of my Lyme disease madness.

Contents

Preface

A boy and his Grandfather are out for a stroll on a sandy beach. Thousands of washed-up sand dollars litter the seashore. The boy hops over each of the creatures in his path and continues forward. The Grandfather continually reaches down to pick up each sand dollar and throws it back into the ocean. The boy asks, "Grandfather, why are you throwing those back into the ocean? There are way too many; you will never save them all, so what does it matter?" The withered old man slowly bends down to pick up another sand dollar, looks the boy in the eyes, saying, "To this one, it means the entire world."

I have always loved the above parable and it is exactly how I feel about writing this book. I understand this material will not be able to solve everyone's struggles in the world, but I know it can assist some. If my journey can inspire and help just one person recover their health, this will surely have been worth the time and effort. I am hoping that one person is you. You have what it takes to overcome your struggles. I know that because you picked up this book. That means that you have a big enough reason WHY and that you are willing to take action. That tells me that you are a fighter, an explorer, a curious soul willing to ethically do whatever it takes to better your life. I understand you are taking a gamble reading this book as I am NOT a doctor, a scientist, nor an expert. I am a regular guy that was tackled by the invisible enemy we know as Lyme disease. Thankfully, I, too, am a fighter and not a victim and I have been able to rise and defeat Lyme disease, thereby reclaiming my life. There is a massive learning curve to heal from Lyme; exploring the many facets of bacteria and their effects on the human body, as well as understanding yourself and your mindset. I am fortunate that I found the time and resources available to put in countless hours of research.

As you know, it is incredibly challenging to comprehend scientific data, studies, and theories while the compounding brain fog of Lyme is suppressing your comprehensive capabilities. Accordingly, I will be limiting the scientific jargon whenever possible. It is as if you are playing a game of bar trivia as the only competitor that doesn't speak the same language, and you are rapidly going deaf at the same time. It is an uphill battle, to say the least. My goal for writing this material is to shortcut the suffering of others. Many of you reading may have been plagued for decades with no resolutions. I can appreciate you have been though many struggles and identify with that. Of course, I cannot make any guarantees or claims that this book is the way to cure Lyme disease. There are many different approaches to healing, and everyone's biology is unique. Also not everyone will apply and take action the same way that I have. That being said, there is a good chance that utilizing the same healing measures that I have taken will result favorably to your own health. All the information I have sifted through and applied over the years will be covered. The information in this book is exactly what has been successful for me, not only in reclaiming my health, but completely revolutionizing and transforming my life for the better. Initially disguised as a dark and maddening curse, Lyme disease turned out to be a blessing.

My hope for you by the end of our time together is that my own perseverance might inspire you to continue the research, continue the fight, and continue the belief that one day you will be fully recovered. This book is not a comprehensive everything-to-know-about-Lyme book. There are far more treatments, methods, protocols, and actions one could learn about that may be useful for some people. The methods delineated in this book are precisely what it took for me to regain my health and well being. I have witnessed others utilize the same approaches with equal results. I am writing from personal experience with the hopes of one day hearing your success story. It will take time; if you have had Lyme disease for a few years or longer, it will not go away in a few weeks. It will probably take a few years to recover. We will focus on incremental positive actions that will compound over time. I feel confident you will see the clear skies of optimal health once again. I wish you success in your journey to health, wellness, and prosperity.

1

CRAWLING OUT OF DARKNESS

Feeling bad doesn't mean your life is shot. A bad feeling means you have successfully identified something that needs to change.

Adventure was all I could think about. I had just finished up recording all my drum parts for the entire album, and I was becoming restless in the unexpected downtime. I certainly should have been napping, but the raw excitement of being finished with recording and new plans for spontaneous adventure surged adrenaline through my blood. The three of us didn't meet until around midnight in Mesa, Arizona. Danny, Storms, and I piled into Danny's orange Wrangler; the engine was still hot from his drive from Palm Springs. We planned to drive all through the night and arrive at the trailhead before first sunlight. The road toward Havasu Falls was slow, dark, and dusty. It took us about six hours to finally coast into the off-road parking lot of the trailhead, arriving only twenty minutes before the sky began to illuminate. We used this time to take a very brief car-nap. I don't know if any of us actually slept. We stepped outside the

Jeep, tightened our hiking boots, strapped on our rucksacks, and began the descent on foot down the rocky path and into the steep, dusty canyon. Havasu Falls is a magnificent location complete with numerous natural waterfalls, stunning vistas, glowing red cliffs, and most notoriously, brilliant turquoise waters flowing over tall chiseled cliffs. It is not only a magical place, but it has a rich Native American history. You can just about feel the native spirit still reverberating between the earthy canyon walls.

Havasu Falls usually is not a day trip. The majority of people will hike in and camp at the falls for a night or weekend and then walk back out. We had the outrageous idea to drive six hours on no sleep, hike the entirety of the trail out and back, then immediately repeat the exhausting drive back to Mesa, all in a single day. It was a ludicrous idea in retrospect, however, we were adventurous and ambitious, and nothing was going to stand in the way of tackling our dream hike. The first half of the day was glorious. We were fortunate to hike under a crisp, sunny November sky with the freshest air one can imagine. We hiked for a couple of hours into the expansively long and narrow canyon and passed the Supai Indian reservation at mile eight – which is known to be the most remote community in the contiguous United States. This village is so isolated that it is currently the only community that receives its mail by postal mule carriers! Continuing a few miles beyond the Supai dwellings, we reached the incredible Havasu waterfalls. We were completely taken back by the natural beauty that flowed before our eyes. We had seen photographs of these falls before, but it is impossible to convey the wondrous experience you can only receive in the physical presence of this magnificent place. The water emits an etherial essence in which photographs struggle to convey.

We were on an adventure high. Not only was it a physical accomplishment to carry your weight out to this location, but the payoff was well worth the effort. Everything had worked out so well. Exploring such a stunning site with great friends, I had almost forgotten about my looming health condition. It wasn't until we turned around to begin the long hike back that I was quickly reminded of the health problems that have been oppressing me for the last few years. The symptoms crept up gradually, and then suddenly. I was panicking; I was so far from any professional assistance. My fear made things far worse. My vision constricted, the brain fog intensified, the dark voices in my head were becoming deafening, my limbs turned numb, the physical pain alarms were getting louder, everything was hitting at once. After years of battling an invisible enemy, (which I still hadn't put a proper name to) I thought I had finally reached the end of the road here in the middle of this vast canyon.

* * *

Twelve more miles of agony; I do not know if I have the strength in me to continue. There isn't a road in sight. There is no reset button that will magically transport us back to the start. Nothing brought us here except for our own feet and an adventurous spirit, perpetuated by the lore of the American Southwest. And now, when I look down, those very same feet that are supposed to carry me out have dissipated into dust. I collapse to my swollen knees; my rucksack slumps over the side, pulling me down to my back. I connect with the dusty canyon floor.

My systems are depleted - like a smoking candle flickering out at the end of its wick. "Everything ends here," I groan to myself. I squint my eyes and stare up at the overarching red cliffs, my vision blurring in and out of focus. The floaters in my eyesight seem to be overtaking my entire field of view, forming their own crowded structures in the sky. I attempt to breathe deep as I wonder if the ancient natives that have dwelled in this vast canyon ever suffered from invisible illness. If so, I imagine they must have believed it to be some form of demonic possession...they wouldn't have been far off. I think about how we equate who we are by the qualities of our personalities, and how that notion has been completely shattered for me now that my affliction has made me an entirely different person; internally dark and mad. With my head resting on a sandy boulder, the last three years of madness and suffering flash through my mind. I simply cannot see past this sad, defeated moment in time. The hope and spirit I have lived my life with have been slowly stripped away and now completely emptied, perfectly depicted by a broken man laying feebly at the bottom of a slot in the earth. "How will I ever crawl out of this canyon? Is there any reason to?"

* * *

This climaxing day in my life was the breaking point. All the physical agony and psychological torture that had plagued me over the last few years seemed to have compiled on my proverbial shoulders to the end; I could carry the weight no further. The worst part was that I had no confirmation as to what was destroying my life. I did not know it was Lyme disease; I had only suspected by that point. Hopelessness is despair, which is the main characteristic of defeat. Defeat, in this case, equals lying down and awaiting death. My illness had destroyed my social skills, lowered my intelligence, handicapped my physical abilities, eliminated my motivation and drive, reversed my positivity, corrupted my memory, and stripped away everything I enjoyed and loved about my life. I didn't care to have, do, or become anything that I had worked for or envisioned for myself and my future. Nothing mattered anymore.

My social skills declining meant that my relationships suffered. New and old connections alike, I could not communicate with the people I used to care about, nor could I make new connections. Looking someone in the eye was out of the question. My brain fog was like a filter on my intelligence, only the basic motor skills would operate, and even those were lacking. There was no way I could solve problems or multitask. The dark, psychotic thoughts that appeared in my mind were chilling and foreign, yet they were in my head masquerading as if they were my own. My physical abilities, such as skateboarding, hiking, rock climbing, and playing music, were severely handicapped. I could not hike more than a few miles without severe joint pain, nor could I rock climb or skateboard to a level I had worked hard to attain. My motivation toward success in the world had been eliminated.

My work ethic declined, which had reflected in my finances. I did not care about my future or anyone else's future that I worked with. I saw the world as a sinking ship, and I was going down with it. My smile had permanently flattened. The glass surely was half empty everywhere I looked...scratch that, it was entirely drained. I could not remember the nature of my relationships, and the memories I did have appeared corrupted. I was unsure of who was actually involved in the memories. Without the history of a relationship, it is hard to operate in the present. The joys in my life had all been stripped away; those activities, people, places, hobbies, items, thoughts, and feelings, have all been manipulated in my mind and I no longer cared about any of them. I wanted out from this shell of meager existence.

Though hopeless, somehow, I thankfully had an ounce of fight still in me; let's call it a divine fighting spirit. All I needed was a point in the right direction. I was always more than willing to do the work if I knew what to do. I can't recall how exactly it happened, but down there at the bottom of the Grand Canyon, I made the decision that I would do whatever it took to find out what was wrong with me and fix it. And so I began the tireless journey that every beaten down soul must take on in order to climb out of the depths of despair and begin the process of rebirth and renewal.

Danny and Storms each grabbed an arm and hung it around their necks. We trudged our way out from the earthly gorge and up the steep canyon trail. Step by pain-filled step, we finally reached the parking lot. As I laid there feeling thankful to be back to the Jeep, I knew I would do whatever it took to feel well again. I was sick and tired of being sick and tired. I would have given anything to get my health back. Nothing else mattered. I did not know that I was about to begin the most crucial transformational journey of my entire life.

2

INTRODUCTION OF MINDSET

When we cannot change the situation, the only way to evolve is to change ourselves.

Most often, we see the world through a single lens, one overall set of views or beliefs that produce the way we think about the world in which we live. Living with disease and illness, that lens that is the easiest to look through would be known as the 'victim-lens.' Looking outward through the victim lens creates a mentality where we say things are happening TO us. We carry the notion that we are where we are in life because of our circumstances, and the bad cards dealt to us. By the time most people learn they have Lyme disease, they are so worn down by the symptoms and the grueling journey of discovering the cause of those symptoms. By then, the disease has already taken full control of their calendars, finances, relationships, and minds. We let Lyme disease define us. We allow it to dictate what we can and can't do. The reality is that our external environment (even our health in this case) does not have to dictate our lives. **We can create our lives based on internal conquest rather**

than external circumstances. When we cannot change the situation, the only way to evolve is to change ourselves.

It wasn't until I changed the lens through which I saw myself that I began to see the circumstances of my wellbeing change. I was able to take a step back and see I had a lot more control over the situation than I thought I did. And you know what is funny? I wasn't the only one suffering from health problems, go figure! It is effortless to get so wrapped up inside your head and dwell on your issues that you forget what is going on around you with other friends and family. This headspace drives despair even deeper. Taking a step back and realizing you are not alone in your suffering can be helpful, though not intended to dwell on others' misery. Just know you are not alone. For me, this crucial lens shift is what spawned my thoughts toward the regeneration of my health. I learned that our thoughts are what produce our actions, and our actions will determine our results. Later a further lens upgrade, taking an even more significant step back after I had regained my health, allowed for the inspiration to create this material in hopes that it can help you or your loved ones.

This informational journey is about overcoming illness, both physically and mentally. Perhaps your journey will even lead you to a full cleanse of body, mind, and spirit. This information focuses on what has worked for me through my journey of overcoming Lyme disease in hopes that it will shortcut your suffering. I know how challenging it is to comprehend words when you have severe brain fog; I will keep the scientific data to a minimum. I think it is essential to include some aspects of each treatment so that we can understand its purpose and how it works, but I promise to keep it reasonably light. For those who need further scientific research, there are plenty of books, websites, case studies, and the like that can give you more scientific details that focus on each topic exclusively.

I encourage you to continue the research on any of the information you find interesting or potentially helpful. None of these methods and principles are unknown. Mostly, I wanted to put together my success story and how it happened so that if it helps just a single person, it will all be worth it. These methods and principles that I have researched extensively and applied have effectively combated Lyme on many people, so I believe this information can help the masses, not just a few. Every human body is different. Every situation and every mind is different, but these are the things that I have studied and used for my recovery toward complete and natural health. Most of these treatments will cost little money and have minimal or zero side effects. The only things you may need to give up is your initial comfort zone and your victim lens (if you have one). If you are like me, I was ready and willing to try anything to get back to being healthy. Thankfully, the following information is just what worked for me and how it could work for you. Today, we crawl out of the shadowy canyon and begin a life that is not dictated by illness. We can refuse to be victims together and let us start to take responsibility for our health.

3

MEDICAL MATRIX

Most late-stage Lyme patients have similar stories. They experience years of a multitude of mild to severe symptoms, attend numerous doctor visits, see all types of specialists, go through countless tests and procedures, and spend a fortune out of pocket. They spend all of this time, energy, and money, producing no answers or, worse, a misdiagnosis. You may even be able to apply this situation to other autoimmune disorders or afflictions; Lyme is not the only one. It is incredibly frustrating trying to navigate the medical system, knowing deep down that the way you are feeling is not normal and having no one there guiding you towards wellness.

There are a lot of fantastic doctors out there. Almost all of the doctors I visited were highly professional and extremely knowledgeable. They were eager to help. The problem is not the doctors or their staff, but rather the system that they operate inside. It is a highly controlled system and regulated by large corporate networks and steered in the direction of profits. Health care is an incomprehensibly massive industry. It is sad to say that when sickness has been cured, the patient is no longer a repeat customer. Do you think big business strategies are designed to keep their clients coming back?

Without going too far down the rabbit hole, it is vital to understand the industry of medicine because that knowledge may affect your future decision-making with your doctor's suggestions. What is essential to understand is that the industry itself controls the information. Pharmaceutical corporations fund research, which unfortunately dictates the direction of the results of that research. Certain natural health methods and principles are not promoted because they do not bring in profits. A natural substance cannot be patented. Usually, if a natural compound is having success in treating or preventing disease, the information is quickly suppressed. The corporations rush to create some synthetic inorganic compounds that might replicate the results of the natural compound bringing with it a long list of harmful side-effects. As we know, our bodies do not function well from inorganic foreign objects. The Journal of the American Medical Association stated that prescription drugs were the third-highest cause of death in the U.S. It is eye-opening when you discover that government is also not for the people when it comes to health, it is for the dollar. Government legislation is swayed by huge corporate lobbying interests and will follow whatever direction the money dictates.

It is equally unfortunate that most medical schools only delineate a small fraction of their medical curriculum on diet and nutritional studies. The reason is that the drug industry has bought the minds of the medical profession. The whole medical education system has been set up and supported by the pharmaceutical industry's major players. Students learn to diagnose and treat a symptom with a drug. When the body has a symptom, it is a warning sign that there is an underlying issue causing harm to the patient's health. If we focus on covering up or eliminating that warning symptom, do you think the patient will become better or worse? It appears that the patient gets better because there is no more cough, no more headache, or no more sinus infection. But what caused those ailments to occur in the first place? Only when we switch our focus to restoring the body's homeostasis and support the natural functions of our anatomy will we see a real transformation of health. The body will no longer be crying out its alarming symptoms, begging us to stop the madness we are putting it through. We can live in harmony within our natural body as it will be strong enough to fight almost anything that comes our way.

The following satirical excerpt about this medical matrix is from a book called *Leadership And Liberty,* co-written by New York Times bestselling authors Orrin Woodward and Chris Brady. "What happened in the late 20's and throughout the 30's [referring to the American economy] is akin to a patient with a head cold getting advice from an over-reactive doctor. Based on some new, exciting techniques just picked up by the doctor at an international conference, the doctor administers drugs that don't treat the cold but make it worse. Seeing this, the good doctor, surrounded and encouraged by other doctors doing the same thing, confidently administers even more medicine. Only this time, there are additional side effects. The doctor, however, doesn't see it that way. Instead, he sees confirmation of just how sick this patient was in the first place and, gee whiz, good thing there's a doctor on the scene to help! Further meds produce more side effects and soon the situation is drastic. Emergency life-support measures are required or else the patient will surely die. The patient is not really living any longer, strapped to the tubes and machines of life support as he is, but he is not dead either. This encourages the doctor and his colleagues to congratulate themselves on keeping such a terminal patient alive and strengthens their resolve to formalize the life-support system. It is at this point that the doctors can't believe their ears when someone has the audacity to suggest that perhaps the patient never needed anything other than a chance to recover from his cold naturally. 'As sick as he is?' They cry, 'you non-doctors are so naïve!'"

By now, you may be thinking, well, isn't the traditional route of treating Lyme disease with antibiotics treating the source and thus removing the symptoms? Isn't that killing off the cause of the illness? I understand antibiotics appear to be killing the Lyme, which is the cause, but what it is also doing is killing the healthy bacteria in your gut and disturbing the body's immune system's natural functions. Our bodies need to maintain that healthy balance of good bacteria. If you do get bit by a tick or perhaps you have the famous bull' s-eye rash, antibiotics can be effective if administered within a short time after infection. In this early stage of bacterial infection, it may be adequate to do a brief round (usually about two months) of antibiotics. Ideally, that would take out the Lyme before it duplicates and fortifies itself into the tissues. A month or two on antibiotics shouldn't wreak too much havoc to the body that it is unrecoverable. Even if this is the treatment you opt for, the following information will still aid in your healing and will build your future-long-term health so that you can truly live up to your maximum health potential.

As we progress through these treatments, you will see a shift from methods of killing the bacteria to the principles reinforcing overall health supporting the body's resistance and repairing mechanisms. If you can master the basic principles, you can master your health. There is a little jingle I hear a lot that goes like this:

> *Methods are many*
> *Principles are few*
> *Methods may change but*
> *Principles never do.*

You will see that you reach a point where you no longer fear your disease when you focus on the principles of health. Fear in itself is a disease. Acting on the fundamentals of a healthy lifestyle gives you confidence and courage, which entirely negates the fear. Can you envision a future where you are waking up in the morning feeling energized, invigorated, and grateful for your life and relationships? Picture yourself in optimum health and feel gratitude at that moment. You did it! You made it through the darkness. Do you see yourself getting out of that bed and standing firmly on the ground, feeling ready to embrace your day? Can you see yourself prepared to march toward a new life full of purpose? You can have this day come. This new era of your life is possible, where you are finally feeling confident with no more pain, no more confusion, no more social anxiety. You can be proud you have made it through the darkness and emerged as a stronger soul, reinforced by a pure body.

4

CONFIRMATION

After much seeking, I found the Lyme-literate doctor closest to me, which was about an hour away from my home. I still wasn't 100% sure what was wrong, but I am very thankful to my great friend, co-worker, and band-mate named Chris, who had the genius insight in thinking it was an immune-suppressing problem. He saw me just about every day for years in which he saw all kinds of different symptoms throughout that time. As we know, Lyme disease is called the "Great Imitator," and it can often make you appear as a hypochondriac. By this point, I had been to over a dozen specialists, had numerous medical tests and procedures, and spent thousands of dollars on costs not covered by my traditional healthcare plan. Because of those experiences and all the research that I had conducted, I already had suspicions it was Lyme by using those clinical case-building methods.

The office I found is called MJA Healthcare in East Stroudsburg, PA, run by Dr. Mikhail Artamonov, M.D. The staff at this facility understood that the ELISA (enzyme-linked immunosorbent assay) and Western blot tests of the modern health care system will almost always give you a negative test result in patients that are in the later stages of the disease. Realizing this was a relief because it was the first medical establishment that took my suspicion seriously instead of assuming hypochondriac and giving a random drug prescription to treat whichever symptom was present that day.

The clinic staff helped me conduct a few different tests, including some different blood panels and a brain cognition test, which covered my head in electrodes and measured my brainwave functions. This test measured spatial navigation, temporal orientation, procedural actions, episodic memory for places, face recognition, and semantic word knowledge. I ranked below 50% in all categories except for spatial memory. That category I scored 100%, which I attribute to my addiction to playing chess to pass the many traveling hours while on tour with my band! Seeing those low cognition scores was intriguing as it quantified my brain fog and declining motor skills right there on paper in front of my eyes. It was a relieving yet sad confirmation of my diminished abilities.

While testing for Lyme, there are a few things you should know about your test results. The test results, for the most part, can be highly inaccurate! They can leave you clues, but very rarely can you be 100% sure of the findings (in the late-stage patients). Usually, if you know you were bitten by a tick recently and you do test positive, then you can be pretty confident that it is accurate. Also, the famous bull' s-eye rash is enough evidence of Lyme disease. If you suspect you have had the Lyme symptoms for a long time now, you most likely will not test positive (according to the CDC's standards). In the late stages of Lyme, the spirochetes have already burrowed deep into the bodily tissue, and also changed forms, escaping the blood tests. So what do you do then? This situation is where you'll hear the term 'clinical diagnosis.' Wikipedia explains this as "a diagnosis made on the basis of medical signs and patient-reported symptoms, rather than diagnostic tests." You will need to examine all the tests and evidence that you have (any Lyme test results, symptoms, blood panels, etc.) and work with a Lyme professional if possible to determine the odds of infection based on all the evidence and probabilities collectively. There are a few other things you can check to point out more evidence of a Lyme infection. For example, there has been new evidence of alterations in the mitochondrial superoxide levels in certain types of cells in Lyme patients. In multiple studies, it was found that patients with Lyme disease have much higher levels than those in the control group. Talk to your Lyme-literate doctor about any other testing and diagnostic methods that they may be using, but it will help the process if you already have some knowledge yourself of what you would like to test.

Opposite of not detecting the bacteria is the 'false positive' result. This result happens when you have another similar infection such as Syphilis that could have cross-reactive antibodies show up on the tests. Either way, if you show a false positive, it means there is something else affecting you and generating similar symptoms. We will discuss the natural treatments that may help lessen or eradicate the illness even if it does not have the official title of Lyme disease. However, it would be wise to keep an open mind that what you have could potentially be something completely different until the evidence says otherwise.

It truly is a massive weight off of your shoulders to have confirmation of an illness that has mysteriously plagued your physical existence. Just stay the course and keep pushing for answers. Due to Lyme disease's resilient cloaking nature, it can be challenging to discern facts from rumors. Because it is an emotional topic for those who have suffered from it personally or seen a family member suffer, it can be easy to jump to conclusions or side with any misinformation that best suits your understanding of Lyme disease. I will be the first to admit that I do not know all the scientific details of the bacteria or the instruments we humans use to discover the microscopic world. I know it can be daunting sifting through an endless supply of information online or in books like this one, not knowing which contradicting articles to believe. In this Information Age, it is easy to become confused. When we have an abundance of information, time is what becomes scarce. I hope this compilation of my research and personal experience will shortcut your research time and thereby accelerate your healing time. I know for sure that I successfully treated myself (and others) by applying the following information in this book: information I have spent years studying, which has saved my quality of life and others who have also found and used the same information. Can you imagine if just one of these treatments or lifestyle changes had the same benefits for you? If you can cut through all the noise of misinformation and rumors and focus on applying a few of these natural treatments and lifestyle changes, I can confidently say it will have a positive effect on your overall health.

5

OZONE

"The possibilities of thought training are infinite, its consequence eternal, and yet few take the pains to direct their thinking into the channels that will do them good, but instead leave all to chance." – Marden

I am grateful for this clinic, and I was thrilled to be starting a treatment specific to the cause. There was indeed hope. Finally, I found someone who recognized the Lyme symptoms as a real problem and had a solution! A solution that did not follow modern medicine's spam-like approach of using a few years-worth of antibiotics leading to a destroyed gut. I immediately got started with the IV treatment. Because this was the very first treatment directed at fighting off Lyme, the initial benefit from this treatment was hope. The importance of this is crucial. If you do not believe you can heal, you will not heal. Read that again: **IF YOU DO NOT BELIEVE YOU CAN HEAL, YOU WILL NOT HEAL!** Author John Maxwell famously says if there is hope for the future, there is power in the present. I just want to stress the importance of our thoughts. Our thoughts can manifest and shape our reality. The more pure your body is, the more accurate that statement becomes. Legendary author Napoleon Hill wrote in his master work *The Law Of Success*, "There is a growing tendency upon the part of the best informed physicians and other health practitioners, to accept the theory that all diseases begin when the brain of the individual is in a depleted or devitalized state. Stated in another way, it is a known fact that a person who has a perfectly vitalized brain is practically, if not entirely, immune from all manner of disease." He continues, "Every intelligent health practitioner, of whatever school or type, knows that 'Nature' or the mind cures disease in every instance where a cure is effected. Medicines, faith, laying on of hands, chiropractic, osteopathy and all other forms of outside stimulant are nothing more than artificial aids to NATURE, or, to state it correctly, mere methods of setting the chemistry of the mind into motion to the end that it readjusts the cells and tissues of the body, revitalizes the brain and otherwise causes the human machine to function normally."

The process was straightforward. The phlebotomist named Asia would put a special catheter needle into my forearm vein that would then be taped to the skin and connected into the IV drip hose. The drip hose connected to a raised tube of water that the ozone machine was distributing the ozone into so that the water going through the IV now had ozone in it as well. Just to note, this tube of ozone water is where she would also mix in the silver hydrosol in future treatments.

In the first treatment session, I developed a strong cough due to the respiratory toxins being stirred up and eliminated from the ozone. This reaction was common, though it slowed my startup dosages. We did not begin with the silver; we thought it best to do a few treatments of just ozone initially to reawaken my body's immune system by the oxidation of the cells.

WHAT IS OZONE?

So what exactly is ozone, and how is it effective against Lyme? Ozone, which has been used medically since the mid-1800s, is so diverse and has so many benefits that it is hard to get a grasp on precisely what it can and should do for you. There are also many ways of using ozone. Let's start with the basics of understanding its properties. Think back to chemistry class if you had one. We all know water is also known as H2O. That simply means it has two parts hydrogen and one part oxygen. The oxygen we breathe is O2, as a single molecule of oxygen always pairs up with another. Well, easy enough, ozone is O3. It carries three parts oxygen. Since the molecular structure already had two paired and balanced atoms, the third hitchhiking oxygen atom is looking for a bond. Ozone travels through the body looking for a way to balance (unload) the extra atom's electrical charge with any other unbalanced charge, such as the Lyme bacteria, other Lyme co-infections, viruses, fungi, molds, parasites, or any other unwanted pathogens.

Not only is ozone terrific at eliminating the bad, but it is also a fantastic blessing to the body. Breathing is the most important bodily function. The human body depends on getting new air almost as quickly as we exhale. Humans can survive a long time without eating or drinking compared to the length of time you can last without breathing. The better the quality of air, the more benefits it has to our bodies. Unfortunately, the industrial age has tainted the air quality, and our bodies no longer are taking in the amount of oxygen needed to have a healthy cellular function. This issue is where the ozone is a significant help. When used correctly, your body will utilize the new ozone oxygen, effectively rebuilding cellular function, maximizing your health potential. Since our cells are mostly water and oxygen, doesn't it make sense to bless the cells with pure water and pure oxygen?

According to renowned medical ozone pioneer Frank Shallenberger, MD, HMD, the single biggest risk factor for disease and premature aging is the way your body utilizes the oxygen. The more efficiently our bodies can use the oxygen intake, the more healing and prevention of disease becomes possible. Without proper utilization, the body produces high levels of free radicals, which the scientific community attributes to be the cause of aging, destruction, and disease. Ozone boosts the oxygen levels in the cell's mitochondria by up to ten times the amount that O_2 can. This oxygen boost creates a fully functional and healthy cell culture while reducing the production of free radicals, thus, once again, preventing early aging and disease.

USING OZONE FOR LYME

As mentioned earlier, there are many different ways of using ozone. Let's discuss just a few options that are most suitable for Lyme. I will point out that each of the following methods can also be used as future disease prevention or routine health maintenance once you are rid of your Lyme ailments and living a healthy life. After reading through these uses, if you feel that you would rather buy your own ozone generator instead of going to a clinic, I highly recommend reading Shallenberger's short book called *The Ozone Miracle.* He covers precisely what you need from a generator and how to use it properly. You do not want to buy a cheap generator off of Amazon for use in your body. You will need a generator made from specific materials so that the ozone doesn't strip the molecules from the device itself. You also want a generator that uses pure medical grade oxygen and not one that tries to make ozone from the air. He refers readers to www.ozonegenerator.com, and you can check out their machines for yourself if that is the route you want to go. They are pricey, but so are countless doctor visits. It helps to start understanding what an expense is and what is an investment in your health.

IV DRIP: The first method we already discussed is the method I used, which is the IV drip directly into the bloodstream. This approach seems to be the fastest most efficient way to eradicate the Lyme spirochetes from the body. The blood travels throughout the entire body, which can deliver the ozone to the hard to reach areas that oral ingestion may not reach. That is the main reason for mainlining into the bloodstream. Lyme spirochetes are very good at burrowing into the joints and organs' tissue, so the IV method can be extremely effective at killing off the bacteria in those areas.

IV INJECTION: The IV Injection is the same function as the IV drip. The only difference is the dosage is smaller in volume but highly concentrated and boosted into the vein quite quickly. This way was the application of choice for a while for a lot of doctors that specialize in ozone treatment. This method has had great success in treating Lyme disease and similar ailments such as ALS and MS. I would like to note that recently a lot of doctors that use ozone treatment have been wary about using the direct injection method because of possible risks. Don't let that alarm you, the risk of any hazards are so small compared to modern healthcare procedures that, in my opinion, it is not even worthy of considering it a danger. The only reason some groups of doctors have been shying away from it is to protect the future of ozone treatments. As we know, medicine is big business for the healthcare companies, and any treatment that threatens their profits will always be under scrutiny. The concern is if something were to happen, the government (who is funded and therefore controlled by big corporations) could confiscate ozone generating machines. I didn't understand this at the time, or I may have done things a little differently. If you want to be a team player and protect the future of ozone benefits for all, then perhaps look into any of the other methods. It may be a little slower, but it is a safe way to go while protecting the big picture for everyone in the future.

DRINKING: We don't need to spend a lot of time here. It is quite simple. I would say this is probably the most common and easiest way of using ozone, especially as a health maintenance protocol. Simply diffuse ozone (at 80 to 90 gamma) into distilled water for about twenty minutes and drink that water within a few minutes after the diffusion. This method is very comfortable for people and still very effective. Another form of drinking ozone is drinking diluted H_2O_2. This substance is food grade hydrogen peroxide diluted in water. I used 35% food grade hydrogen peroxide and started mixing five drops twice per day into a tall glass of water, working my way up to thirty drops. I continued for a few weeks then tapered back down to a few drops to complete the protocol. This treatment has many health benefits equal to ozone since it also has an extra molecule of oxygen.

SAUNA: If you are near a clinic that offers an ozone sauna, this can quickly fast-track your healing. Consistent use of saunas has many health benefits, especially for heart health, and when combined with ozone, it becomes quite the powerhouse treatment. If you have the funds and space, you can purchase your own personal ozone sauna, which could do wonders for your long-term health. Either way, if you get the opportunity to use this treatment, it could help eliminate Lyme via the use of the ozone. Because of the effects of the sauna, it would boost the overall immune system giving you even more of a fight against illness.

10 PASS: The 10 pass is quite a similar process to the IV drip treatment. It is essentially the same for a patient's experience. You would sit for an hour and a half or so with an IV in your arm. The difference of this method is your blood is taken out, diffused with ozone, and then returned into your bloodstream. That may sound like a scary process, but it is actually a routine modern medical process. There are two main methods of this treatment. You would do one or the other, depending on the facility's equipment, but both achieve the same results.

The original method is known as Normobaric. This way uses gravity to pull the blood out and gravity to push the blood back inside. You can probably visualize how it works; the bag is held below your arm to withdraw the blood, ozone is gently diffused inside the blood bag, and the bag is held above your arm using gravity to replace the blood. The updated method is known as Hyperbaric. During the Hyperbaric process, your IV connects to a machine. Instead of utilizing gravity, a vacuum pulls the blood through the device, which then mixes in the proper amount of ozone, as well as an anticoagulant to prevent clotting. The blood and ozone mixture is vigorously shaken up and pushed back into your body, delivering the ozone into the bloodstream and distributed throughout the body. The positive hyperbaric pressure protects the red blood cells during the extreme shake-up process. Another benefit to this machine is it can make the process quicker for the patient. One potential drawback could be any adverse reactions a patient might get with the anticoagulant. If you think it could be a potential problem, the medical staff can let you know which brand they use before deciding how you would like to proceed.

The 10 pass method uses more ozone than the other methods; however, there is a debate on whether it is more effective than the direct injections. The discussion says that even though the 10 pass is higher ozone content, it has already used some of its potency on the blood outside the body as opposed to the injections having a more potent effect directly in the body. Either way, they all have documented tremendous results with Lyme disease and many other diseases. You will have to research the applications and prices that are best for you. Your treatment method will be dictated by the equipment and practices of the facilities nearest you unless, of course, you are willing to travel.

If you have been suffering from Lyme for a couple of years or longer, you may want to consider buckling down and finding the money for a few ozone treatments, at least, or ideally a complete ozone protocol. I would say out of every treatment I did this was the best one to start with, which is why we are starting with it in this book. There are many other ways of using ozone, and for a multitude of different reasons, however, you don't need to get overloaded with the details. We covered enough to get you started or at least enough to jog your curiosity to want to research more about the impeccable properties of ozone.

To bring it all together Jacob Swilling, Ph.D. research scientist says it best in his book *Medical Ozone:* "Regular use of ozone therapy strengthens the immune system by enhancing circulation, providing an oxygen-rich environment for cellular rejuvenation, cleansing the blood of impurities, clearing plaque from the arteries, optimizing the acid/alkaline balance of the body, improving nutrient assimilation and by removing putrefactive deposits from the intestines and colon. These and many other beneficial results of ozone therapy make ozone ideal for rejuvenation and life extension and perhaps the most effective means for reversing the 'aging process.'"

6

COLLOIDAL SILVER

After a few ozone treatments, we began to add the colloidal silver into the ozonated water. We were using the brand Argentyn 23, whose colloidal silver product is called Bio-Active Silver Hydrosol. I looked forward to each treatment session as I could feel the results. The treatments took about two hours, depending on the volume of silver. I used this time to de-stress and clear my mind. I was in a small room, usually by myself. The phlebotomist would hook me up to the IV and then give me space, checking in now and then. This process was a great time to relax, de-stress, meditate, and envision a healthier future-me. Occasionally, there would be another patient in the room, which I found pleasant. It helps to hear someone else's story, a fellow warrior on a similar crusade. Lyme disease can leave you in a very dark and lonely place within yourself, and talking to others about it can help you resurface from the depths of inner despair. Sharing ideas and other knowledge that has helped each other is also a great way to gain insight into what else is out there. Ah, the power of a like-minded community! You may find it helpful to join a Lyme meet-up group in your local town or perhaps an online forum community. However, in-person meet-ups can be far more beneficial. You may even build life-long friendships out of it.

WHAT IS COLLOIDAL SILVER?

It would help to understand what the word means before understanding what this treatment can do. A colloid is a mixture containing insoluble particles suspended in a different substance. More relevantly, we are talking about colloidal silver, tiny positively-charged silver ion particles suspended in water. Colloidal silver is one of the most potent natural antibiotics ever discovered, and it comes with zero side effects when used correctly. Our bodies already have and use silver even without ever supplementing it. That means that it is not a foreign object to your body. Silver properties are anti-viral, anti-bacterial, anti-fungal, and anti-pathogenic. It has tremendous results in seeking out, binding, and killing the Lyme bacteria and co-infections. Unlike antibiotics, the silver is also effective with viruses, yeast build-ups, and fungal infestations. Both fungus and yeast have been a growing problem in our society, and thankfully silver is highly effective with Candida and other types of parasitic life forms infesting our bodies. A modest dilution of just five parts per million is enough to kill off any known microbe in under six minutes. The other great thing about colloidal silver is because it is in the colloidal suspended state, it gets absorbed into your system before it can get to the intestines. That means that it does not kill off your environment of healthy bacteria as antibiotics do. Colloidal silver is tasteless, odorless, available to buy, easy and affordable to make, and completely non-toxic.

Another benefit that colloidal silver has that antibiotics do not have is healing capabilities. Yes, just like ozone, silver is great at attacking enemies as well as being a blessing to your body. According to Dr. R.O. Becker, a well-known and respected biomedical researcher, silver is known to promote bone growth and accelerate the cell growth of healing tissue by over 50%! Continuing research on the benefits of colloidal silver, you will find it boosts your immune system immensely, helping you fight off the yearly cold and flu season. Silver can transport high levels of oxygen into your system, up to ten times its atomic weight. There are even many new studies lately showing evidence of silver damaging cancer cells.

Are you starting to see the potential that these treatments offer? They are combative and effective at ridding Lyme bacteria, viruses, and other maladies, and they are a blessing to your body at the cellular level, in more ways than one. Think of it like we own a dilapidated, run-down rental property, and the condition of the property keeps bringing in bad tenants. We can evict them for not paying rent or for trashing the place, but the next tenants we bring in are just as bad. With these homeopathic treatments, we are evicting the bad tenants while fixing up the property, adding value to attract a new and improved situation, free of deadbeat tenants (and no more late rent checks!).

USING COLLOIDAL SILVER FOR LYME

Using colloidal silver for Lyme will be very simple. If you are doing an IV drip of ozone, it can be at the same time through the same solution. This is the method I did, and it was tremendously worthwhile. It also saved some time by treating with ozone and silver in the same session. You can also do an IV drip of just the colloidal silver without any ozone. You may find this is a more common option depending on where you live. Do not worry if you are not near a clinic that offers this. The most common way to use silver is simply to drink it. Usually, the recommendation is to put the colloidal silver under your tongue for thirty seconds and then swallow. Doing this allows it to enter your bloodstream more directly. It is straightforward to start a protocol with one teaspoon the first day and then work your way up to ten teaspoons throughout the day. Depending on how severe your symptoms are, you may want to continue around ten teaspoons per day for a few weeks or until the symptoms start to disappear. Scale back down to two teaspoons per day for a maintenance dose after you feel you have succeeded with the heavy dosages. Once again, you want to wean into the more substantial quantity dosages to avoid the Herxheimer reaction (also known as a healing crisis). Your body needs time to remove the garbage out of your system. It takes time to evict bad tenants. Give yourself time to succeed.

You can also put colloidal silver into a brown glass spray bottle for other applications. This way, it can be pumped up your nostrils or sprayed into the mouth toward the back of your throat for any cold or sore throat symptoms that pop up. It can also be sprayed into the air in front of you so you can breathe the vapor through your nose or mouth and into your lungs. Spraying can help diminish any coughing, sore throat, or sinus issues you may have.

Silver Hydrosol is not very expensive compared to other supplemental remedies, though, you may want to look into how to make it yourself. If you are just looking to get over your symptoms as fast as possible, I recommend buying it and beginning immediately. However, once you see how amazing colloidal silver is, you will most likely think about using it long term; in that case, it would be worth researching how to make it yourself. I recently bought 16 ounces of Silver Hydrosol online for approximately $80.00. In Max Crarer's book *"Everything You Need To Know About Colloidal Silver,"* he shows you how to make colloidal silver for under $3.00 per liter. I want to point out that the high quality of a professional silver product will most likely be most effective. However, for long term maintenance use, the colloid you can make yourself will be adequate to maximize your long-term health.

SAFETY

If you are like me, when you first heard of putting silver in your body, you were very skeptical. It did not sound right to me, mainly because I was ignorant of it. In other words, you don't know what you don't know. When I thought of silver, I only pictured jewelry or my grandmother's eating utensils. I did not know that silver is a trace element found in a natural diet. Colloidal silver has been used medically for over 100 years. Injections especially have been documented with tremendous testimonies.

As we learned earlier, effective homeopathic remedies are always under fire from mainstream media and corporate propaganda. The opposition with using silver still flaunts the stories of the few cases that state a patient turned blue (picture a Smurf) from using silver in their body. Let these articles only offer you a laugh, as that is all they can offer. Every case of turning blue has proved to be photo and story manipulation by the media, or simply the person consumed an absorbent amount, well beyond the recommended dosages. Even the high doses we discussed are not even remotely close to quantities used in those few cases. Not one person has ever been reported ill or dead from properly using colloidal silver. It would be wonderful if we could say the same about pharmaceutical medications; unfortunately, the list of side effects for a single pharmaceutical drug could be as long as this paragraph. You will see for yourself just how safe and secure it is to begin a colloidal silver protocol.

* * *

I can remember driving home after the fifth treatment and feeling incredibly normal. In this case, normal was awesome! I hadn't felt that normal healthiness vibration in years. The mental fog, which was my most tormenting symptom, was slowly lifting! The opaque vail I had barely been surviving beneath was finally tearing. I had a higher consciousness, and I had energy. Inner peace had replaced the tense anxiety. I could tell the treatments were piercing the Lyme disease stronghold! The storm clouds were finally lightening up. I continued this IV process consistently for another two months after that until I started tapering down to one treatment a week and even every other week. I wanted to continue going, but paying $250.00 each session was adding up very quickly. I could tell the IV treatments made a tremendous amount of progress already. I thought I could continue tackling the rest of the Lyme through adjusting to a healthy lifestyle and beginning some other homeopathic protocols that I had already heavily researched.

7

LYME DIET

I never imagined that one day I would write a book, especially a book that includes a section about diet. I was the kid eating fast food almost daily, drinking public water directly from the faucet, mixing Sour Patch Kids into any dessert possible, and sneaking into dumpsters at 3 am to take the garbage bag of leftover pizzas from Cici's restaurant. I did not think twice about consistently eating fast food. One November, I even decided to eat at McDonald's for every single meal of that month. Many of these habits and tastes that built up as a kid still carried over into my young adult life. Also, I have spent a lot of my time with Lyme disease while on the road touring around the country, and as you might know from being on road trips, it is tough to find healthy food on the go. It would have been wise to use grocery stores and stock up on fresh foods, but when you have a whole band and crew in the vehicle, you usually have to go with the group consensus, which was often the easiest and fastest option: fast food or gas station food. Gas station food became so commonplace that my buddy Danny and I would sarcastically refer to ourselves as "gas station wine connoisseurs."

You can start to see what I mean when I say Lyme disease has been a blessing. If anything, it was a huge wake-up call. To be honest, I wouldn't have changed if it was any less crippling. My problem needed to be severe, or else my stubborn self would never have changed. It is interesting how we laugh and joke about our poor health choices until our good health no longer exists. I now fully understand that overcoming these substantial obstacles in our lives truly makes us who we are. Or, on the contrary, we can let the obstacles define us. But we both know you and I are more resilient than that. It just takes a higher level of thinking, combined with action and persistence. Do you feel like you are at a breaking point in your health? Ask yourself, is it worth experimenting with altering my diet if it could mean potentially feeling much better than how I usually feel? If you are thinking this way, then let's begin making some significant changes.

I do not intend for this chapter to be like normal diet books. Usually, those are hyping some trendy, well-marketed variation of an existing diet. Some famous examples of this are the Keto diet, Paleo diet, Flexitarian diet, Vegan diet, and many others that have become more popular recently. Ideally, this chapter will leave you with a guideline of what has helped me significantly. I will try to keep it brief so that we do not hype it up more than we have to. This content will not be spelling out details on specific food combinations, and there surely will not be any meal recipes (though I think some of my friends would tell you I can make some tasty broccoli tacos!). Instead, the following information is once again focused on a few core principles. This way of eating is fantastic at eliminating or reducing symptoms and is probably the fastest protocol in this book that you can apply to feel results almost immediately. You can apply as much or as little as you want to, and again, do your own research for your specific situation. Food is one of those things that people get very protective about, and if that is you, then you may not like this chapter! I have found to get any fruitful results in anything requires taking actions or establishing habits that we may not like. Usually, it takes a massive awakening to want to change any eating habits. I am thankful this was the case for myself.

First and foremost, I focused on removing the most symptoms as fast as I possibly could. I struggled with multitasking, writing, recording, and performing music, and I did not know how much longer I could hide my poor performance, not to mention my poor attitude among my friends and family. I had to cut through the fog as fast as possible. I believe this lifestyle tweak will do the same for you too. Here is the main principle with this Lyme disease diet. The whole focus is to reduce inflammation. Inflammation is aggravating a lot of the symptoms that we experience with Lyme disease and other ailments (joint pain, coughing, brain fog, and fatigue, just to name a few). If inflammation is causing a lot of those symptoms, do you think it makes sense to remove inflammatory foods from our diet? I do not know how, but this made a lot of sense to me at the time. This knowledge was the beginning of my understanding of some of the human body's systems as a whole.

DAIRY

The first alteration in my diet was eliminating dairy completely. I had been consuming dairy my entire life. I never realized how many foods actually contain dairy. Once you start looking at ingredients in the foods you are buying, you will see dairy is in practically everything! Okay, not everything, but it is in a lot of unexpected foods, especially pre-packaged foods. Recognizing this was a challenge at first and somewhat overwhelming. It will take time to learn which foods are dairy-free, and I can assure you that it does get effortless after reading most of the food labels. Give yourself time to learn. The good news is, the age we live in there are more and more foods coming out as dairy-free. My first few trips through the grocery store probably took a couple hours or more. Now I breeze through the isles as I know what I am going for, and the other foods are just distractions. After the learning curve, it makes shopping a lot easier since most of the grocery aisles will not have anything for you. There will be a few main isles which will have your best dairy-free foods, and then, of course, the produce section will be an essential department for you.

So what is it about dairy that is harmful? As I mentioned, it promotes inflammation in your body, but what does that actually mean? The more you research dairy, the more evident it becomes that it is plain and simply not healthy for anyone. There is enough research out there by reputable people that I can say that confidently. The only reason you may have doubts is because the dairy industry is one of the best industries at marketing their products and controlling the research. There have even been documents that went public with correspondences between the dairy industry leaders discussing the leverage they have for future sales if they can indoctrinate children at an early age of their lives. Creepy, I know. These corporations are purposefully targeting your children and teaching them it is healthy to consume dairy when the fact is you will find plenty of research that confirms the opposite. You do not need milk for strong bones; in fact, it is the exact opposite. Milk weakens your bones and promotes osteoporosis.

The human body likes to maintain a neutral pH balance. That means a balance between acidity and alkalinity, although if I had to lean toward one side, it would be alkalinity. There is a lot of new research on the benefits of having an alkaline-rich diet, showing that disease cannot survive in an alkaline body. I need to do more research on this myself. Dairy is an acid-forming food, which means your body must compensate for the increase in acidity whenever you consume dairy to restore a neutral pH balance. Your body does this by taking the reserve of alkaline in the form of calcium, potassium, and magnesium, which are stored in your bones. You can imagine what this does to your bones! With these minerals leached out of your bones, they are more susceptible to fractures, which is quite the opposite result of what milk is supposedly doing for us. You will learn that countries with the highest rate of osteoporosis also have the highest dairy consumption.

What's more, tests have shown that dairy protein known as casein (which is 87% of cow's milk) is a significant factor in cancer growth. One of the best resources for scientific research on dairy is a book called *The China Study* by T. Colin Campbell (Ph.D.) and Thomas Campbell II (MD). This book is filled with scientific data proving the malicious effects of dairy. Below is an excerpt from a section where they studied the "protein gap" in less developed worlds, and what they found was incredible. They looked at how carcinogens in the body promote cancer growth with diets containing dairy compared to diets not containing any dairy. "What we found was shocking. Low protein diets inhibited the initiation of cancer by aflatoxin, regardless of how much of this carcinogen was administered to these animals. After cancer initiation was completed, low-protein diets also dramatically blocked subsequent cancer growth. In other words, the cancer-producing effects of this highly carcinogenic chemical were rendered insignificant by a low-protein diet. In fact, dietary protein proved to be so powerful in its effect that we could turn on and off the cancer growth simply by changing the level consumed. Furthermore, the amounts of protein being fed were those that we humans routinely consume. We didn't use extraordinary levels, as is so often the case in carcinogen studies. But that's not all. We found that not all proteins had this effect. What protein consistently and strongly promoted cancer? Casein, which makes up 87% of cow's milk protein, promoted all stages of the cancer process. What type of protein did not promote cancer, even at high levels of intake? The safe proteins were from plants, including wheat and soy."

These findings are not just the case with animals, by the way. Throughout the book, there are more than enough studies involving humans for decades of their lives, proving the same conclusions. I could go on and on quoting this book, and others like it, but this is hopefully enough to get you thinking and to begin your own research. Just watch out for industry-sponsored research. How can the dairy industry get away with lying you might be wondering? There is something known as scientific reductionism. The company that funds the research is usually looking for a particular spin on the data. Most of the time, the data is zoomed in too far to tell the whole story, or manipulated to create a different narrative. This constructed narrative designs to bring trust to the product along with more profits to the industry shareholders. Unfortunately, in the world that we live in, profits come before health and nutrition. If you are genuinely suffering from your poor health, I will encourage you to try a month of eliminating dairy from your diet. What do you have to lose?

GLUTEN

The casein protein in dairy has a very similar molecular structure to gluten, and roughly half of the people who are casein intolerant are gluten intolerant. The very same week I cut dairy from my diet, I decided to cut out gluten. At first, I had some challenges because this led to me not eating many carbs right away since I was new at finding foods that did not have wheat. I avoided grains all together for a while. It was not wise that I tried hot yoga for the first time during this hearty dietary shift. My body was practically in what is known as ketosis, which is where it burns ketones (which are from fats) for energy instead of the usual sugars (carbs convert into glucose). Ketosis happens a few days after not eating any carbs or if you are fasting. My body could not handle those changes combined with the intensely heated room and paired with the fast-paced yoga movements. After only ten minutes, I felt myself blacking out and about to faint, so I quickly laid into child's pose to avoid collapsing. After that experience, I took it a little slower. I realized it might take some time for my body to adjust. I started to slowly replace those carb-heavy foods such as pasta with gluten-free foods rather than cutting them out completely. Some of my favorite go-to meals were wheat-heavy, and I was bummed about cutting them out. I know now that it is very simple to eat the same types of food if you want, you just have to find a gluten-free version of it or make it yourself with any grain substitutes. I use organic rice flour or coconut flour a lot, even corn or quinoa flour substitutes are quite common now. I do not trust the mass-produced corn, so I do try to limit those foods. Unfortunately, a lot of the gluten-free substitutes are corn-based. We would not have as much to pay attention to if GMO farming did not take over the food industry, but once again, profits over nutrition.

A gluten-free diet has increased in mainstream popularity as far as diets go, and I have been thinking a lot about this. Why is gluten-free on the rise? Is it because of the new GMO wheat product recently manufactured that is now affecting humans? Or has this always been making people react, and people just did not understand it until recently?

If you start diving into information attempting to answer these questions, you will most likely come to similar conclusions that I have myself. We are at war with corporations that mass produce modified crops while using harmful chemicals such as herbicides and pesticides for us to ingest. Unfortunately, at least in the United States, our farms have been acquired by huge corporate interests, including food titan Monsanto. Monsanto was recently bought by pharmaceutical giant Bayer, which seems to be a perilous conflict of interest. Bayer can now sell you foods that make you sick and then treat you with a manufactured drug to mask the symptoms in an endless cycle of expensive biological destruction. Monsanto has patented crops designed to grow despite the dense herbicide sprays that rain over them. Monsanto owns a product that most people know as a weed killer called Roundup. You can buy this at any garden store to kill off the weeds in your lawn. What most people might not realize is this is what is sprayed on their food as well! The design of these modified crops is to grow amidst this chemical spray, but we humans are not designed for such poisons. One of the most dangerous ingredients in Roundup is Glyphosate. Glyphosate has been under scrutiny lately, as it should be, as well as Monsanto in general. Glyphosate has recently proved to cause cancer by a US court case and causes many other issues that affect the human body. This issue is not just the case with wheat, but wheat is probably the most susceptible to soaking up the chemicals and transferring it into your body. Other non-organic crops will still contain chemicals and should be avoided as much as possible. Eating organic produce is the best chance of reducing pesticides and herbicides from getting into your system.

The sad bit about this situation is this; when farmers use Glyphosate products, they think they are doing their crops a service by saving them from bugs and animals to produce a better yield. What can happen over time (within five years or less) is the land becomes so infertile it is hard to grow anything! Often, farmers will have to move to a new field or do a lot of maintenance to produce a yield the following season. Plants have their own self-defense mechanisms in place if you grow them properly. When the soil is fertile and thriving with the proper nutrients that the crop requires, the plants will produce defenses that keep predators away. The soil needs an appropriate PH level along with balanced levels of calcium, magnesium, potassium, and other nutrients, and it will flourish all on its own, without manufactured chemicals.

The food will be healthier and taste significantly better too! The exciting thing about weeds is that they grow in exact locations for a specific reason. Usually, if you see a cluster of weeds growing, it is because that area of the soil lacks magnesium. Ironically the weeds are there to help balance out this deficiency. Unfortunately, most weeds get poisoned rather than carrying out their purpose, which destroys the soil at the same time. The weeds are a symptom of a systemic issue. Just like our biology, if those symptoms get covered up, the real problems continue to grow.

All in all, gluten can affect individual people. Perhaps, a lot of the people who benefit from cutting out wheat are actually feeling the benefits of cutting out the chemicals such as glyphosate. More studies will have to occur to know for sure, but until that time, if you want to reduce your symptoms, you are probably best to cut out wheat and other GMO crops completely. Over time it may benefit you in doing some tests, trying 100% organic and non-pesticidal herbicidal wheat, and monitoring how you react. That is something to strive for, no matter what foods you are eating. I would hope that the meals are as natural and pure as possible. We are what we eat, right? I continue to avoid gluten/wheat as much as possible, even after a few years of feeling great. It may be fine going back to organic wheat, but I have no incentive to risk it. Mainly because once I start eating wheat again, I know I will end up eating foods that are using these GMO chemically saturated crops (it is hard to know when out to eat in restaurants). I would rather avoid that risk altogether. Yes, you will probably have to pass up the office Christmas party cookies or the tray of wedding hors d'oeuvres that pass under your nose, but with a little self-control and a lot of conviction for what you will put in your body, it will get more comfortable and easier to eat well and recover your health. I know I am never going back.

PLANT-BASED DIET

"Americans love to hear good things about their bad habits." - T. Colin Campbell

Now being totally aware of my dietary intake, it was only a matter of time before questioning the rest of my usual consumption. It did not take long for me to learn to continue cutting out the rest of the animal parts I was eating. As a Lyme disease sufferer who was actually on the up-and-up, this was the next best step to elevate my healing. First, I had cut out only red meats, which is a great place to start. Eventually, in about another six months, I had eliminated all animal consumption.

For any of the serious candidates reading this that want to improve your illness suffrage, this may be the most challenging chapter to read. We have covered dairy and gluten, but those are minuscule now when we are talking about eliminating (or changing) our main dish! You may be asking, what are we going to eat?! Meat has a much stronger hold in our dietary lives than gluten or dairy as it is usually the main course or mixed into almost every dish in some way or another. I can tell you this: my reason 'WHY' is more significant than my desire to eat meat. Once I made the decision, it was easy. I have not gone back once and do not miss it. The only animal product that I eat very occasionally is eggs if it comes prepared in an entree in a restaurant (I love Drunken noodles from Thai restaurants and it is usually in that). For the most part, I would say my diet is about 99% plant-based.

So I had a big reason why...what is the reason that Lyme sufferers might want to consider switching to an all plant-based diet? There are a few reasons. Very similar to dairy, red meat is inflammatory. Inflammation exasperates the Lyme symptoms. There is a time and place for the body to use inflammation for good. Unfortunately, this chronic inflammatory response that our bodies have to the relentless feeding of these causative foods builds up and creates immobility, pain, confusion, depression, and many more ailments.

Red meat is extremely tough on the body. Our system needs to work overtime to try to break it down and flush it out. Over time, the consumption of this flesh gets stuck and builds up in our digestive tracts and becomes rotten from the inside out. To add insult to injury, this creates a perfect environment for Lyme spirochetes and other parasites, including roundworms, tapeworms, yeast, and others. That is another positive attribute about removing meat from your diet: you reduce the potential for pests entering your body and weaken those already residing within. Most known worm parasites feed off the flesh and often found in pork, fish, and beef (yes, even in developed countries). We will cover this more in-depth later, but know that you are reducing potential threats by not eating meat. These threats include antibiotics, carcinogens, pharmaceuticals, GMO feed, diseases, fattening agents, rogue meat parts, steroids, viruses, and bacteria that are all found in various fleshy products; the mass-production meats and poultry are the worst of the animal products.

Lyme disease can have a very random and mysterious effect on human biology. It can create chaos, especially with your immune system. Lyme disease can actually alter your biology, which, as mentioned before, can change who you are as a person. That was a scary revelation for me in the beginning as I felt my personality darken. The results of numerous studies show having Lyme disease for a long time can create an allergy to red meat. That means that even aside from all the potential toxins that animal products can bring in, your body may be triggering an allergic response to the ingestion of red meat. Having Lyme disease and continuing to eat meat could be equivalent to someone who is severely allergic to cats and continues to go over to pet them and rub their face in the cat fur. The result of how this person would feel after petting the cat is obvious.

If you have applied everything we have covered on diet to aid your healing process, you would be considered gluten-free and vegan. That is the shortest way I have found of categorizing my diet to other people. Veganism has a lot of stigmas attached to that label. It is funny you will start to hear the same responses from people, usually just out of ignorance. I say that kindly, ignorance is not stupidity. We don't know what we don't know, and frankly, before I had a reason to do any research on it, I had the same mindset, which is once again why I am thankful for my Lyme disease. We, as young and growing humans, do not question how we are raised. We take the food that is given to us, thinking that is what we need. It is comical; before when I ate the average American diet no one cared what or how I ate. As soon as my transition to vegan, all of a sudden people care about my protein intake! That is usually the main question I get; "What do you do for protein?" And my answer is always a short explanation: that the same protein we get in meat derives from the protein in the plants and grains that the animals eat. Also important to note, high levels of protein does not constitute a healthy diet.

Let's take a sidebar here for a minute to get a brief understanding of what protein is all about. There are hundreds of thousands of different kinds of proteins, and they are the essential building blocks of our bodies. They are chains of amino acids, and they can act as hormones, enzymes, tissue, and many other functions. These die out over time and need to be replaced by eating more proteins. The protein in plants is known as "low-quality" to mainstream nutrition. Still, one could find enormous amounts of research that confirms that the healthiest type of protein is the plant proteins, which synthesizes these proteins slowly but efficiently. The human body will manufacture all the correct amino acids from plants exclusively. You will get more than enough good protein by eating a plant-based diet. I would like to say something about that too. I am wary about the high volume of protein intake recommended. We have this push for heavy protein consumption diets, but then there exist diseases like Parkinson's and types of Alzheimer's that patients have a massive buildup of protein in their brains. Isn't it strange that those diseases are not common in countries with a "protein gap"? In the book *The China Study*, the two author-scientists make a very comprehensive case against animal proteins. They studied this topic for almost all of their careers, and they conclude that animal proteins are the triggers for cancer, heart disease, and many other illnesses. They show consistently that "nutrients from animal-based foods increased tumor development while nutrients from plant-based foods decreased tumor development."

Another stigma, let's call it a myth, surrounding veganism is that it leads to malnutrition and a weak body. There are plenty of people that would shatter this myth who are fully vegan and competitive bodybuilders. One example of many I could give is a man named Patrik Baboumian. Patrik is a world record holder and known as Germany's Strongest Man (2011). Looking at him, you would never guess he only ate plants. With biceps that wouldn't fit into a regular tee shirt, Patrik is one-hundred percent vegan. There are ways of being an unhealthy vegan, of course. Eating a diet heavy in the frozen meat substitutes and sugary junk foods could lead to malnourishment. That is why I like the diet classification of 'plant-based diet' over vegan; it is a little more telling. We need those life-sustaining fruits and vegetables, raw and uncooked as much as possible. When we cook the veggies, it changes the molecular structure, especially in the microwave! The microwave will destroy any nutrient structure of the foods, so you may want to stay away from it (If you are a visual person, look up the Kirlian photography of plant energy). I usually try to steam the vegetables in a pot when I do cook them. If the majority of the food in your shopping cart is from the produce section of the grocery store, you are on the right track!

Since mentioning Kirlian photography and energy, there is one thing I would like to point out. After removing meat from my diet, I have become aware of a stronger connection with animals. I care about the lives of the animal kingdom just as much as the human species. I have never been much of an emotional or empathetic person; however, that has changed significantly.

It could be from removing dead negative animal energy from my body or purely detoxing and flushing debris. Or maybe it is from decalcifying my pineal gland (see the chapter on pure water). Nevertheless, I have a deeper connection to life than I did before I started this health crusade. I can feel external energy and tune in to higher frequencies of thought. If you have not experienced this you may think I sound insane now, but that does not change its reality. It is not a rare day when happiness and appreciation are swelling throughout my body. I can't say it is from eliminating meat precisely; it could be just a surge of wellness from generally feeling good and recovering. Either way, it feels good having that growing connection to life!

This chapter has been most challenging to write about as it swims upstream to many societal strongholds. My health challenges have led me to pull the handcuffs off my preconditioned wrists and learn that I can swim upstream. I believe we have diet and nutrition very wrong in our society. I also think animals have the right to live without being sacrificed for our pleasurable consumptions. I know that belief alone challenges a lot of people. It is just a conviction that has developed throughout my journey. I do not want to come off as pompous or arrogant. I respect your right to make your own decisions. I hope whatever action you take leads you to an abundance of health and wellness while at the same time promoting health and life (rather than death) for you and the other humans and animals in your life.

If this plant-based diet chapter interests you, I encourage you to read *The China Study*. The book gets a lot of criticism as it directly attacks two huge industries, so I recommend reading it for yourself if you want more scientific data. We could go on and on in this dietary arena, but I don't want to overwhelm you with pushing veganism to you. That is honestly not my goal. I purely am showing you how it has dramatically increased my wellness, and I am trying to just scrape a little information off the top of the vast ocean of dietary-information. We are leaving so much out, but I think you get the point! If we want different results, we need to take different actions. With obesity ever-increasing, heart disease rising, the diabetes community growing, autoimmune disorders evolving, cancer rates climbing, we know that living the normal conventional way of life (at least in America) while expecting good health is a tall order. If the research strongly shows that diet and disease are linked, and all of those rising ailments are normal, then I believe it is in our best interests to start being extremely abnormal with our diet!

DIGESTIVE ENZYMES + PROBIOTICS (LEAKY GUT)

Gluten can have such a disastrous effect in the body and usually traced back to something known as 'leaky gut.' This malady was first recognized as a real problem by homeopathic healers and nutritionists and lately getting a lot more attention from the mainstream. However, your family doctor will probably tell you not to be concerned. Standard medical facilities will not recognize it until it is studied in med school, and it might be a while until that happens. I hope nutrition is first recognized in med schools as crucial to health, and then maybe from there, things like leaky gut would be studied. I found out about this through my iridologist. Perhaps you know, but I didn't realize what iridology was initially. According to Wikipedia, iridology is "an alternative medicine technique whose proponents claim that patterns, colors, and other characteristics of the iris can be examined to determine information about a patient's systemic health. Practitioners match their observations to iris charts, which divide the iris into zones that correspond to specific parts of the human body. Iridologists see the eyes as "windows" into the body's state of health. Iridologists claim they can use the charts to distinguish between healthy systems and organs in the body and those that are overactive, inflamed, or distressed. Iridologists claim this information demonstrates a patient's susceptibility towards certain illnesses, reflects past medical problems, or predicts later health problems." Yes, some people may consider it pseudoscience or what have you, but either way, my iridologist knew I had Lyme disease without me telling her, just by looking at a close-up photo of my eyes. She also enlightened me to leaky gut, thereby recommending some treatments and dramatically adding value to my healing. It also opened another door of understanding as to how the body's digestive functions work. I did not even consider that this could be an issue before our meeting. It helps just to learn, even if it seems irrelevant at the time, and maybe some more dots will be connected in the future.

The idea behind leaky gut is this; due to increasingly high levels of chemicals and toxins in our food and high levels of sugars and heavy alcohol consumption, over time, the stomach and intestinal walls develop tiny holes in the protective lining. These small holes are large enough for undigested food particles to slip through and enter the bloodstream. After these particles are in the blood, your body sees them as foreign objects and sends a response to combat them and attempt to eliminate them from your system. You can probably imagine the baggage that this places on your immune system! Many medical professionals believe this to be the main trigger for autoimmune disorders such as Crohn's disease, Lupus, fibromyalgia, arthritis, allergies, and many others. Frequently in our illness, the body can never catch up or keep up to heal itself because it is overworked by processing all the food we tend to over-consume and the foreign bodies in our systems such as chemicals and unnatural GMO foods. Leaky gut turns some of those ingested particles into poisons, penetrating directly into the bloodstream and carried throughout the body. That's why it could potentially be causing symptoms where you might least expect it. It is a systemic issue, meaning, dealing with the entire system.

Understanding all that, you are probably starting to understand how leaky gut could go hand in hand with Lyme symptoms. It is a perfect storm. We need a robust immune system to combat the Lyme bacteria, and the leaky gut could be sending the immune system troops into a different battle. Imagine if you could eliminate that distraction how much more effective your fight against the Lyme bacteria would be. There is a way to rebuild, but it takes time. So in the time that it takes to rebuild, the best thing you can do to alleviate your symptoms is to stop ingesting the foods that act as poisons, the main one being gluten. Now, you might explore and find that organically grown local wheat is better for you and run with that. But to jumpstart your healing, it may be best to eradicate all gluten, at least while you rebuild and then slowly experiment with organic, non-GMO wheat.

To rebuild from leaky gut issues, most homeopathic practitioners tell you to do a few different things. The overall principles are as follows; focus on removing the inflammatory foods in your diet, rebuild the healthy bacteria in your gut (also known as fauna), and help digest your new foods more efficiently. We have already covered the importance of removing inflammatory foods. To create a healthier bacteria culture, look into daily probiotics that you can take, either as a supplement or a beverage. I took a brand called Jarro-dophilus AF. This brand does an excellent job of keeping their probiotic cultures alive in the capsules for delivery into your system. Oh yes, if you didn't know, probiotics are living cultures, known as 'good' bacteria. It will take time to rebuild this fauna, but consistent daily habits will get you there.

Adding to this, it will help to give aid to your digestion. As I said, undigested food particles that slip into the bloodstream are the main problem with leaky gut, making sense to boost the process of breaking down the food particles. I took digestive enzymes from the brand Nutramedix in powder form, twice a day, taken with the probiotics. This remedy can be taken simultaneously with any of these other supplement protocols we cover in this book as they are focused on rebuilding your body. The ultimate goal is not to need any supplements eventually, so what we are doing is supplementing the processes your body lacks at the moment, due to the Lyme or other illness or poor lifestyle. We can enhance long enough until your body is doing the work all on its own, as designed. Once again, give yourself time. Your body can heal; you have to trust the process. Digestive enzymes and probiotics should help issues you may be having that are adding on to your illness. It is hard to tell what is going on when you have a mix of symptoms. Still, chances are doing this simple protocol will boost your body's ability to heal itself and eliminate any potential symptoms that are adding on to your illness.

8

SAMENTO + BANDEROL

Lyme Disease's most-feared opponents: Samento and Banderol. Two cunning warriors that work together like Odysseus and the Trojan horse. Personally, these two have been the best all-around additive treatment (rather than a subtractive like fasting or diet alterations) to combat and eradicate the Lyme bacteria, clearing away the symptoms even further at a fairly substantial rate. As an overview of these two herbs' functions, I use the analogy of Samento being Odysseus, Banderol as the Trojan horse, and the Lyme bacteria being the city of Troy. As you may know, the spirochetes have many different forms and bond together in what is known as a biofilm. This biofilm creates a fortress (Troy) that is impenetrable initially by your weakened immune system. If you know the story, you know the Greek warriors built a humongous wooden horse as a "gift" for the stone-walled city of Troy. Troy opened its gates and wheeled the splintery structure inside the walls, praising it as a gift to Athena, the Goddess of War. Inside the belly of the wooden horse were over thirty Greek warriors led by Odysseus, waiting for the city to rest. As the city slept in the dark hours of the early morning, the Greeks climbed out of the horse, opened the gates for more soldiers to enter, and began to destroy the great city of Troy from the inside out. This attack is precisely what happens on a daily protocol of these two supplements! The Banderol breaks through the biofilm, exposing bacteria vulnerable to an attack by the Samento from inside their walls!

Samento is a pentacyclic chemotype (that does not contain tetracyclic oxindole alkaloids-or, TOA free), of the vine Uncaria Tomentosa, commonly known as Cat's Claw Creeper, (Cat's Claw for short) with reported antibacterial and antiviral properties. Cat's Claw is a tenacious vine that grows mostly in the Amazon rainforest. Cat's Claw got its name from its hook-shaped thorns that act as claws on a limb. These claws carry the vine up the tallest tree trunks to the forest canopy to maximize exposure to the sunlight. It is quite amazing watching time-lapse videos of this vine clawing up the trees; you see it taking on quite a cat-like personality. Banderol is known to have antibacterial, antiprotozoal, and anti-inflammatory effects. It is from the bark extract of a tree called Otoba that grows in the similar South American regions as the Cat's Claw Creeper. Thankfully, both of these remedies are well known medicinal herbs, and extracts are easily obtained online or at local natural health stores.

A study by the Lyme Disease Research Group at the University of New Haven shows microscopic images of Lyme bacterial cultures and their aftermath of mixing in different antimicrobial agents. They show the control without any agents; the Lyme is flourishing and safely thriving within their biofilm; the image is a lively green cloud. Next, they show a slide with the traditional Lyme medicine known as doxycycline. This antibiotic killed off only one of the three (known) forms of the Lyme, the spirochete, and it actually expanded the colony size of the round body form bacteria. The slide looks like the first image, but the green cloud is spread out and has claimed a wider territory. Third, they show the colony introduced to Samento, which killed off a considerable portion and disorganized the colony; however, some live cells remained. This slide's image looks like a small condensed green paint splatter. Next was Banderol, which killed off ninety percent of the culture but left its size the same. Picture the image of the first slide, but instead of green, it is orange, signaling a mostly dead but same sized culture. Lastly, and thankfully, they introduced both Samento and Banderol, Odysseus and his Trojan horse, into the bacteria. Looking at the slide image, you would think they forgot to upload the picture. It is a blank slide with a few scratch-like hair-thin lines. No cultures or remnants exist after being introduced to our two steady warriors.

The report states, "Samento and Banderol had significant effect on all three known forms of B. burgdorferi bacteria in vitro. We have also demonstrated that doxycycline, one of the primary antibiotics used in the clinic to treat Lyme disease, only had a significant effect on the spirochetal form of B. burgdorferi." That is the reason why most modern healthcare patients will relapse within a short period of time, only to return again and again for more antibiotics. The study continues, "The other very important fact needs to be considered for an effective treatment for Borrelia infection: this bacterium typically has a life span ranging from several weeks to six to eight months; therefore, it may take six to eight months for even one generation of Borrelia to become exposed to the antimicrobial for elimination. Since the herbal extracts like Samento are reported to be nontoxic, they can be safely taken daily for the long period of time necessary to thoroughly eradicate Borrelia from an infected body. In summary, our study has provided in vitro research data on a novel treatment approach using herbal antimicrobial agents to efficiently eradicate B. burgdorferi, the Lyme disease bacterium."

I say this is the very best all-around additive protocol for Lyme Disease for a few reasons. Using these two antimicrobials is affordable, easy, portable, safe, discreet, and extremely effective. At first, Samento and Banderol's tinctures might seem expensive, but compare and contrast their costs to that of the IV treatments or even just buying organic fruits and vegetables. I used the Nutramedix brand for both Samento and Banderol, and I continue to buy them as a liquid in the 2 oz bottle. At the time of this writing, you can get the 2-ounce Samento on Amazon for around $70.00, and the Banderol is the same price. These will probably last you about a month or two. The good thing is the cost will not be long-term. As the study above inferred, I would give it six to eight months of using it every day, two to three times a day, and then start to wean off or reduce your dosage over the next couple of months. This usage will cover any potential dormant forms of the bacteria, and it will give your body a chance to fight them in its entirety. So for a six-month protocol, you are looking at around $840. I have helped some people where this is the only protocol they used aside from healthy living, and all of them got their lives back on track. If your total investment in healing yourself and getting your life back is less than $1000, I will count that as a significant return on investment!

The Samento-Banderol protocol is pretty pleasant compared to some others. All you do is put drops of each tincture into a cup of water and drink it. Simple. It does not taste bad; in fact, I have grown to like the taste. If this is the first remedy you are attempting to combat Lyme with or if you are still heavy on symptoms, you will want to wean into the protocol. The goal is to drink around thirty drops of Samento and thirty drops of Banderol in the morning and then again at night. Start the first day with three drops then add a drop each day. You could add a third dose in mid-day if you want to attack it hard, but I warn you that it may have some repercussions. There is a reason for weaning into it drop by drop.

First, your body needs time to remove the dead waste that these warriors are killing off. Picture bodies stacking up at the front gate of the walled city of Troy. That is why doing some kind of cleanse or detox before this protocol is beneficial as it clears the body's garbage pathways. As you increase the drops, the bacteria will be killed off faster and in larger quantities. Again, this can lead to what is known as a Herxheimer Reaction. That reaction produces an effect that creates increasing Lyme symptoms temporarily until the waste flushes from the body. For example, if you suffer from brain fog, as I did, your Herxheimer Reaction may be a brain fog that is twice as powerful. Or maybe your joints ache worse than average. Usually, it will take the symptoms you often have and temporarily magnify them until your body eliminates the waste.

Most people I know that used Samento and Banderol correctly and consistently all have had tremendous results. The biggest challenge you may face is getting through the initial first few weeks. Stick with it, know it will get better for those that stay the course. Those who stay will be champions! Once you feel like you have made significant progress, you could experiment with scaling down your drop amounts. If you feel suitable for a few days at half the dosage, then it is probably fine to do half the drops. If you start feeling symptoms arising, ramp it back up. That is the beautiful thing about this protocol. You can adjust it in real-time, as you feel it necessary. You can bring it with you anywhere and take as much or as little as your situation requires. As you are weaning back off of it, you will probably be clear of symptoms for a few months, but I would circle back to do a maintenance protocol every three months for a while after. I went the entire last year without taking any and with no symptoms resurfacing. Being happy that I was feeling excellent, I still decided to do a month-long protocol to make sure no stragglers are waiting in the shadows. After overcoming your symptoms, this is a terrific protocol to come back to if you ever get bitten by a tick again. To this day, I am very thankful for stumbling across the information that led me to give Samento and Banderol a try. I hope your results are equally as successful!

9

PURE WATER

Water is the driver of nature. - Leonardo da Vinci

It is one of the most abundant substances in the universe, and yet it could very well be the most misunderstood! It is the reason civilizations have clustered since the beginning of time. Its very presence will hold rival animals at peace while they congregate in the dry African deserts. It is the great teacher. Its molecules that we see today are the same that were here since the beginning. It is energy; it is wisdom; it is the driving force of life; it is water. Water is the critical building block of nature and all living creatures. Because of its abundance, we tend to overlook the secrets and the God-like nature that water holds. As water is the essential building block for life, this chapter could potentially be an essential building block in your quest for health. Understanding the power that pure water can have on your overall wellness is crucial so that you may have a big enough reason to change up some old habits that may be feeding disease. By the end, you will see that water plays a vital role in your body, mind, and spirit.

THE PROBLEM

Once known for its automobile manufacturing plants, the city of Flint, Michigan has recently developed a new persona. If you occasionally see the news or follow current events, then I would bet you have heard of the Flint water crisis. In 2014, Flint switched their tap water supply from Lake Huron to the Flint River to save money. Unfortunately, the Flint River is heavily contaminated and toxic, far beyond the water treatment facility's reach. This poisonous water swirling through their outdated lead pipe infrastructure created a deadly tonic delivered right to Flint residents' faucets and drinking glasses. From the time of the water source change until it switched back, there were a few deaths and many people hospitalized for diseases and chronic health problems, including lead poisoning, legionnaires disease, infertility, behavioral problems, and many others. The water source has switched back in Flint; however, more questions developed about the rest of the country. Flint's water crisis spotlighted a problem for the entire country. I only hope the light is bright enough to create the change that is absolutely needed.

The above paragraph is an extreme example of a real problem. It has opened our eyes and begun a line of questioning on whether our water is safe or not. I think it is terrific these talks are finally happening, though, we are still a long way away from turning on the faucet and filling up your cup with drinkable water. You might be thinking that you drink from your tap all the time, and it is fine! I hope you come to understand; this is about playing the long game. Drinking impure water will not have any noticeable effects short-term unless it is at Flint levels. But over time, day in and day out, you have debris building up and solidifying in your body's systems. The total dissolved solids, the chemicals, the heavy metals, the bacteria and viruses all enter your bloodstream and happily distribute throughout the body.

The poor quality water situation in most of the world is a challenging one. There are plenty of communities that struggle day by day even to find or have access to water of any quality. Thankfully some great organizations are utilizing new technologies to solve a lot of those problems little by little. Many communities throughout the world that have access to water have given control of water to the government to tell us what is safe to drink and to control how the water is delivered. Yes, I am blessed to live in a country that does not struggle to have access to water and am grateful for that. And it is nice that we can have water delivered with the effortless turn of a faucet, but can we trust the quality of that water enough to drink it? Unfortunately, as we first saw in Flint, the answer is a resounding no!

The Environmental Working Group (EWG) did a study lasting over three years and found that 85 percent of the population's drinking water contained, on average, 316 contaminants – of which 60 percent of these have no safety standards and no regulation by the government's Environmental Protection Agency. The EPA has not updated their standards on whether a chemical is harmful at specific levels since 1974! Think of how much we as a species have learned about the human body and how many new technologies and processes we have developed since 1974. Your local water "safety" reports are using extremely outdated standards to tell you your water is drinkable. All that said, it does not even truly matter what the standards are. We are a surviving species that is intelligent enough to know that any lead, arsenic, pharmaceuticals, fluoride, pesticides, chlorine, or radioactive waste will not be good for our bodies. Let's briefly go over some of the top contaminants found in the public water supplies.

Lead: As you are probably aware, lead made a popularity spike as a contaminant when it was found to cause brain damage to children that have eaten paint chips, as it was a main ingredient in paint. We have since eliminated lead paint from the shelves, but the lead problem is worse because it is a primary contaminant in the water supplies. Along with developmental disorders and brain damage in children, even low doses in adults can cause high blood pressure, memory loss, fertility issues, and even mood disorders. High levels of exposure can cause anemia, kidney problems, brain damage, diseases, and early death. Thankfully, lots of lead piping infrastructure is swapping out with better materials; however, even in those new delivery systems, it is still in the water through other means, such as trash dumps, industrial waste, etc.

Arsenic: If you have seen the T.V. show *Forensic Files* or any other crime shows, you probably have heard of arsenic. I would often hear of it during the two-hour drive home from working in New Jersey. Chris and I enjoyed listening to the audio of *Forensic Files* on SiriusXM satellite radio. Arsenic has been used redundantly as the murder weapon of choice in many cases as it is a slow and almost untraceable poison. In those many unfortunate murderous tales, usually, the victim is given such a minuscule amount of arsenic in their food over a few months. Throughout this period, the victim gets incrementally sicker day by day as the poison builds up in their system. Their symptoms closely resemble a mysterious terminal illness which looks to be natural causes, unless the forensic team has a suspicion of foul play and tests the hair follicles for arsenic. They usually can tell almost up to the exact day when the poisoning began. Quick *Forensic Files* spoiler, it is often the spouses of the victims doing the poisoning! Arsenic is a natural metalloid chemical that is very poisonous. Beginning symptoms of arsenic exposure include stomach pain, vomiting, diarrhea, impaired nerve function, brain fog, declined motor skills, and many more. In the persistent cases of long-term poisoning, the symptoms intensify until incapacitation and then death. Even at fractions of those lethal levels, I personally just would not want any of that in my system.

Chlorine: This chemical element is most often a water treatment method of choice. That means the facilities are purposefully adding this to the water. While this chemical kills off a lot of the bacteria, it is also slowly killing humans. According to the U.S. Council of Environmental Quality, people who drink chlorinated water are 93 percent higher at risk of developing cancer than among those whose water does not contain chlorine. Not only does it increase the risk of cancer, but ingesting chlorine can lead to heart and liver problems and a laundry list of smaller, yet chronic issues throughout the body. Historical fact, chlorine was used in its gaseous form as a chemical warfare tactic in World War I. Chloramines are also a significant water contaminant, which forms when ammonia mixes into water that contains chlorine. Chloramines are usually added as a secondary disinfectant. When mixed in with naturally occurring materials found in the water supply, chlorine and chloramine create disinfectant byproducts (DBP's), which once again cause cancer according to laboratory testing.

Pharmaceuticals: You probably would not take your grandmother's heart medicine, or your uncle's diabetes shots, or even use your friend's eczema creams unless of course, a trusted medical professional prescribed you one of those drugs. Most of us do not want to risk taking pills that come with extreme side effects unless we absolutely have to (according to a doctor's recommendations). If that is true for you, then I think it is safe to say you would not want these manufactured chemical compounds in your body whatsoever. Unfortunately, for most of the U.S., this is a growing concern. The U.S. Geological Survey conducted a study in 2000 which found one or more medications in 80% of the water samples drawn from a network of 139 streams in 30 states. They found substantial levels of antibiotics, antidepressants, blood thinners, heart medications (diuretics like hydrochlorothiazide, calcium-channel blockers, digoxin, ACE inhibitors), and hormones (testosterone, estrogen, progesterone), and painkillers. The water treatment facilities currently do not filter out all of these contaminants. In 2013, the EPA put out a similar report confirming findings of over 25 pharmaceuticals in the 50 largest water treatment plants. Mitchell Kostich, the EPA research biologist who led the study, commented, "We were surprised to find that many drugs occurring across all the wastewater plants. We were also surprised to see so many drugs of a particular class—the high blood pressure medications—appear at those levels across the board." While many officials would argue that these are trace amounts that would not cause any physical effects, think of what long-term exposure could do built up throughout a lifetime, especially as they start mixing and creating unstudied chemical concoctions.

Furthermore, if the problem is not controlled now, it will continue to grow to larger and larger proportions of contaminants as companies continue to put out more drugs for more symptoms. The Mayo Clinic stated that over 70% of Americans are already on medications of some kind. Not only will these contaminants affect humans in the long run, but according to the FDA (surprisingly), it is already affecting aquatic life such as fish and plants, even at the trace amounts detected. That is a challenging situation as the chemical and pharmaceutical companies have a firm grip on the lawmakers and water safety guides. It will take a significant movement to get restrictions put in place for making any kind of change to the water supply.

Fluoride: Fluoride (sodium-fluoride) is a neurotoxic chemical that officials say we need in our water and toothpaste to prevent tooth decay. While there is fluoride found naturally in the earth, the substances dumped intentionally into our public water supply is unfiltered waste products of the aluminum and fertilizer industries. Proponents of fluoridated water use narrow-focused research to make the case that drinking fluoridated water reduces cavities and tooth decay in children and adults. Is this chemical put into the drinking water supply to reduce tooth decay? Just think about that for a minute. Why would we put this chemical as "medicine" for a specific purpose into the drinking water? How can you be sure you are getting enough or not ingesting too much? Why don't we put other vitamins in the water? It does not make any sense. Do you think our bodies would create a body part that relies on an outside chemical? Nature is smarter than that.

Fluoride is one of the most controversial topics when discussing water filtration because the misinformation on fluoride is abundant. There are plenty of people that will give you outdated information saying that tooth decay rates decreased once fluoride was added to the water supply. That is a myth because dental hygiene simply became better and more frequent at the same time, which is why those tooth decay rates dropped. Surprisingly, even The World Health Organization (WHO), which is usually in favor of fluoride, released data showing tooth decay rates have 'precipitously declined' in all the western countries, even those countries that have not been using fluoridated water. Even in the more progressive countries that have already abolished fluoride products, the tooth decay rates have not increased since the abolishment. With consistent ingestion, the symptoms of fluoride can start to show in our society. A large scale study published by the National Research Council stated fluoride toxicity causes side effects such as skeletal fluorosis as the first sign, including muscle wasting and neurological damage, and Alzheimer's and impaired nerve functions in the brain. Also, joint and bone problems occur, such as arthritis, osteoporosis, bone fractures, stiff joints, deformities of the spine, cancers, and calcification.

The process of using sodium-fluoride in the water supply originates back to the early 1930s. Major manufacturing corporations like Alcoa were looking for a way to remove the toxic byproduct as it was injuring thousands of factory workers from exposure. The industry crafted a very successful public relations campaign to spin the narrative about the safety and benefits of adding this to the water. Yes, the same product used as rat poison would be sold and added to the water supply. Dr. Dean, who was with the National Institute of Health, was a strong voice for fluoride safety. Not surprisingly, he just also happened to be a major shareholder of the Alcoa company. Dr. Dean later admitted (in court under oath) that he was incorrect when he originally published that fluoride was safe and yielded dental benefits. The American Dental Association or any other government organization responsible for water safety never acknowledged Dr. Dean's admission.

There is a vast conspiracy with this topic, and you will need to do more research yourself. Please understand, the controlled opposition is powerful. A simple internet search on the subject will bring you an assortment of sites dedicated to promoting as well as others challenging fluoride. Even if you eliminate the possibility that this could be a conspiracy of the industry to gain more profits, or as many groups think, to dumb down the population to submit to government control, it is looking for a solution incorrectly. If we are trying to prevent cavities and tooth decay, rather than add chemicals into the water, have we stopped to consider if our high sugary, toxic diets may be the culprit? Since most dental professionals agree teeth utilize fluoride from topical application rather than ingestion, it makes sense to avoid drinking fluoridated water altogether and brush your teeth with fluoridated toothpaste. That way, you will put it into your teeth without ingesting too much of it into your body. I do not touch the chemical at all, even with toothpaste, and have had no tooth decay. Eliminating poisons from the shower is my next step!

PURITY

***Pure water is the world's first and foremost medicine. –
Slovakian Proverb***

As we eat, drink, or breathe, we take in substances that our body will either use, store, or eliminate. The body will use only the organic minerals that we consume. Plants can convert inorganic minerals to organic; however, the human body is not capable of that process. So what happens to all the inorganic minerals in a human body? If the body cannot flush them out efficiently, then these minerals get lodged in our bodies. By drinking water filled with these harmful substances and chemicals, it is impossible to flush out as we keep bringing in more. If the body cannot assimilate those foreign minerals, it will begin depositing them throughout the body. A perfect example of this is a kidney stone or gallbladder stone. Deposits in the joints give arthritis, calcium buildup in the heart leads to heart failure, in the blood creates hardened arteries, and throughout the skin and other vital organs, it is evolving the aging process and disease.

Water is a solvent. Pure water can dissolve these solids that have built up throughout the body and eradicate them. Over a lifetime, the average person will consume over 450 glasses filled with a combination of these solids. Picture how that might affect your system. If you can stop adding new deposits in your body while also breaking down and removing the old, you will witness a look and feel of age-reversal like you may have never experienced before. It is like taking out the garbage of a cluttered house! We bless the cells in our bodies when we consume pure water. It is comparable to an automobile engine. We are to flush and change the oil of a vehicle every so often. That is because, over time, rust or sludge or dirt will build up in the engine oil (the blood) and needs to be filtered and purified with new oil. Like the engine, the body needs that lubricant pure and clean for it to operate efficiently.

I am sure in the back of your mind, or maybe fully consciously by now, you know you should have the highest quality of water possible for maximum health. So what can be done about this? Do you ditch the tap and buy bottled water? Do you bring in an expensive filtration system? After years of studying private water company's quality reports and filtration methods, there are only a few bottled water brands that I will drink when I am out on the road. Most of the leading water bottle brands are just selling close-to-tap quality water or product enriched with some unnatural process. I stay away from major brands such as Nestle or Aquafina. You can buy a TDS meter at a low cost to get an overall idea of how much debris is in the water; however, it will not pick up on chemicals like fluoride. Whether you are buying water or looking to control your tap water, there is one play that you can bet on and be sure you are getting the absolute purest water that nature intended: distilled water.

DISTILLED WATER

There are many different types of water. You may have come across many of them, including snow water, rainwater, hard or soft water, boiled water, etc. The very best, most pristine type of water you can use is distilled water! The mechanics of distilled water is quite genius. It is nature's chosen method for cleansing her living waters. Since you reside on planet Earth, you must already know how this system works. The sun evaporates the groundwater, which turns into a vapor rising into the sky, leaving behind all of the polluted waste that mixed in the water. In the sky, the vapor turns back into water droplets forming rain clouds. Once the water droplets are too heavy for the cloud, the rain falls to the earth once again. That does not mean you should go out and consume rainwater in the cities. In our modern-day, the rainwater starts perfectly pure but is quickly contaminated after falling through the polluted air and mixing with other toxins along the way.

Distilled water is the best natural solvent. It will dissolve food particles and break down the nutrients delivered to the cells or wherever they are needed. Not only is water a solvent and a regulator of temperature, but water is also a transportation system. It can deliver nutrients in plants and animals as well as carry out the garbage. In the same way it can transport nutrients up a stem or through a vein, it can also deliver unwanted debris and pathogens if it is not pure. That is where distilled water is perfect for the job. It is entirely neutral, not carrying any baggage with it. It can attract and transport essential nutrients as well as sweep up the inorganic compounds and flush them out of the system. Once again, the body will use the organic minerals; all others must leave or stay in the body. Distilled water will dislodge, break down, and transport these foreign inorganic compounds out for good. The organic materials will remain in the tissues and then utilized. It is stunning seeing the disastrous effect polluted water and food can have on our biology. This miraculous substance called distilled water will produce longevity in many ways. Many people even consider distilled water to be the long sought after fountain of youth.

There is an oppressive myth that acts as a gatekeeper to the logical conclusion that this pure water would be suitable for our health. The opposition states that distilled water will produce poor health and malnourishment, as it will leech the minerals out of your body. While this water is fantastic at transporting debris, it is only carrying out the inorganic and leaving the organic nutrients in your tissues. There is a popular article you can easily find online titled "Early Death Comes From Drinking Distilled Water." This story is a wholly fabricated article by an organization that sells reverse osmosis machines, which is ironic as R.O. water is very close to distilled water. There are no dangers to drinking this pure water, only risks to drinking impure water. The other debate is that there are no minerals in the distilled water. That is just silly as we get most of our essential nutrients from natural food or from our own body manufacturing them within itself (during a long water fast). All the adverse claims against this magnificent liquid are usually scam artists or companies with an agenda to sell other devices. There is no scientific basis concluding adverse effects from drinking distilled water, only the opposite.

PINEAL GLAND

Your body is an incredible conduit of energy and consciousness. The human body is a magnificent system that works symbiotically; all processes working together for a complete system. But what is in the driver seat of this superb machine? From where do our thoughts and actions come? I believe it is important to think about these questions to begin to understand the body's potential. I would like to pause the scientific outlook here and turn to philosophy. I believe this is important to think about from a different perspective. I would like to go on record right here and mention that what I am about to discuss is not all proven or even 100% my philosophy, though I do subscribe to the wonder of it all! I think there are many missing pieces to the mainstream religious narratives of who we are and where we come from, or the teachings are heavily encoded so much that we just do not comprehend.

You might think that our individual thoughts and actions come from what we call our soul. The soul is the misunderstood essence of the source of who we are, with or without the human body attached. The well-known French philosopher, mathematician, and scientist René Descartes believed that the pineal gland is the "principal seat of the soul," and also the origin of all of our thoughts. The pineal gland is a tiny pinecone-shaped gland stuck between the two hemispheres of your brain. It is also known as the "third eye" in eastern philosophies. Mainstream science initially told of this gland being responsible for melatonin production and regulation and some other chemical processes like supplying the DMT for dream creation. Many scientists have been coming around to the idea that this tiny grain-of-rice-sized gland has a lot more to it than we can see, mainly in the spiritual arena. Water has a significant effect on the pineal gland, as you will see in the next section.

CALCIFICATION

Over years of drinking and bathing in toxic water, eating a poor diet, and living in many other modern-day contaminants, the pineal gland in the brain becomes calcified, or in other words, turns to stone. Due to deposits of calcium, fluoride, phosphorus, and other toxins, it becomes hardened and dormant, solidifying the gland and rendering its physical and spiritual functions cut off from the rest of the brain. The pineal gland is also known to be the regulator of time. It is my personal theory that time seems to go faster and faster as we get older only because our pineal glands become less functional as it becomes solidified with poisons. We also let ourselves forget the art of living in the moment. The pineal gland is a sponge that soaks up these foreign chemicals, especially fluoride. Usually, you can see this gland in a skull X-ray of an adult as it appears the same as a bone in the image. This gland is so profoundly affected by the toxins we intake because the blood-brain barrier does not isolate it. In fact, it has very abounding blood flow, taking second only to the kidneys. You can imagine any toxins traveling through your bloodstream could pass through this tiny gland and stick in its sponge-like tissue, building up its hardened structure. The good thing about this unprotected blood flow to the gland is that it works the same with decalcifying, or reversing the calcification. When using distilled water in your body, it will purify the blood, carrying out toxins. Distilled water is the very best solvent. Switching to distilled water will start a lively river flowing through you and will wear away at the calcified walls encasing the pineal gland.

When you begin drinking only pure distilled water and removing toxins from your body, you start the process of decalcification. Depending on your age and the water that you have been drinking your whole life, it will most likely take a few years or more to break down deposits in the pineal gland. Consistently drinking over a gallon of distilled water every day will slowly erode the buildup and begin transporting the waste out of the body. People that stick with this process have shared similar testimonies of the pineal gland reawakening. With the pineal gland coming online, people will experience what is known as a crown chakra burst; they see a brilliant white light in their head. They see this beautiful white light not with their eyes, but with this new sensory gland that has been sleeping all their lives. This experience is also known as Kundalini rising. Meditation practices focus on pulling the body's electric energy up the spine into the crown chakra, or the third eye pineal gland. Perhaps that is the same white light in the tunnel that people commonly report during a near-death experience. That light is said to be the soul, seated at the pineal gland, which is the inner eye that can see this brilliant ball of energetic life-light. Could our entire essence be this ball of light? Are we a star in this body of flesh and bones? The white light is just the beginning of the reawakening. This tiny gland is said to be the conduit for transmitting and receiving divine information. Awakening the gland can produce divine consciousness, clairvoyance, telepathy, intuition, oneness or global connectedness, and enlightenment, among other attributes.

Modern western medicine declares that the human pineal gland forms on the 49th day of gestation. Coincidently or not, eastern medicine holds that the soul incarnates into the body on the 49th day of gestation. If it is true that our soul is the essence of who we are, and our soul is a ball of light, equal to a star, it does not seem like a coincidence that the day the 'stargate' gland is formed is the same day that the 'star' arrives. It is said that water is the lubricant of dimensions, connecting the physical world to the astral plane. Interestingly, a baby is completely submerged in water (it is actually amniotic fluid, which consists of fetal urine; urine is mostly distilled water) throughout this gestation period, including that significant 49th day. Whether this is reality or not, it is enough to make you think! Though our physical realm has a lot of afflictions, the circumstances of life are quite amazing! I believe French philosopher Pierre Teilhard de Chardin when he famously said, "We are not human beings having a spiritual experience; we are spiritual beings having a human experience."

What does all this have to do with Lyme? If the goal of all of your efforts is to feel better and reclaim your life, then I believe this is all extremely vital to the success of that venture. We are imprisoned in the notion that health is only relevant to the physical being. Modern-day science is finally agreeing that wellness is a complete package of body, mind, and spirit, all coordinating energy beyond what we can physically see. Considering any potential healing capabilities of the spiritual part of you may potentially go a great distance for your physical health; it surely has for me. When I say spiritual, I do not mean pertaining to religion, but actually, the spiritual energy that encompasses your body. Some people might refer to this energy as your 'higher self.' To reiterate, if you want to reap the many benefits of drinking pure water like your body is built with and designed to use, you will have to control your own situation. The repeating message of this book - you cannot put your health into the hands of the government or other institutions. If you want your health back, it has to derive from you.

HOW TO HAVE PURE WATER

I hope that my over-philosophical-emphasis on the importance of water made some sort of impact in your mind as it has for me. Water has such amazing spiritual and physical properties that it is easy to get carried away in the subject. I believe drinking only pure water will be one of the most beneficial changes you could make for your health, whether you have Lyme disease or not. Commitment and consistency are key; it is easy to fill a glass of water from the tap when you are thirsty. That was the majority of the liquid I drank throughout my life before receiving the blessings of pure water. It will take a little extra effort to set up a system for clean water, but the time and money investment will be well worth it. As the information before this shows, I am obviously passionate about drinking distilled water only. If this is all you are interested in, just skip over these other filters. However, if this is not viable initially, other options will at least reduce the larger contaminants, some better than others. I progressed through each type of filter one by one, using them for a while before upgrading. There are many different ways of filtering and treating your water at home. Some filters mount straight to the faucet, some sit on the counter, others install under the sink, and entire house units treat the water as it enters the house, usually in the basement or a utility closet. In case you are not aware, let's briefly go over the most common filters.

Carbon filter: This is the most basic filter. These are the faucet mounts or the filters commonly built into refrigerators. Carbon filters block larger particles like sediments and silts. If the filter is activated carbon, it will do a good job of removing foul odors or discoloration from the water. It is satisfactory at making the water appear to be drinkable. These filters are affordable but usually need replacing frequently. The downside of these filters is that they do not remove the chemical contaminants such as fluoride and chlorine, and the same goes for the heavy metals such as lead. Brita is a popular carbon filter brand. I have used a top-loading filter called ZeroWater, which had a more elaborate 5-stage filter system that worked well but was expensive to replace the filters every few weeks.

R.O. filter: Reverse-osmosis water filters are the next step toward water purity. Usually, these filters will have a few different stages, the first being the activated carbon filter. What makes these R.O. filters so different is at some point in its filtration system, there is a semi-permeable membrane that allows the water molecules to pass through, which will stop a lot of the micro-contaminants that the carbon filters cannot. An effective R.O. filter can filter particles up to .001 microns in size. That is quite remarkable! Reverse osmosis is the filtration method used by the U.S. military, as it is the most transportable way to obtain pure water. The price of an in-home R.O. filter has dramatically fallen in recent years.

You can get a great setup installed under the sink for just a few hundred dollars. And if you have minor handyman skills, you can easily install it yourself to save some money. I bought an under the sink system from a company called APEC on Amazon and it is a terrific product. While this is one of the best ways of obtaining close to pure water, it does have some drawbacks. Once again, filters need to be changed, although usually not as frequently, which cuts down on your costs. I change my filters once a year. Also, there is a tendency for bacteria to build up inside the filters over time. If the R.O. filter isn't filtering as it does when it is new, you could have a large volume of that bacteria get through to the other side. These filters can also leave your clean water with an acidic P.H. level. It is best to have either neutral or alkaline, but acidic R.O. water is most certainly better than drinking all those contaminants of the original tap water.

Distilled water: Nature's perfect purification process is easily replicated and achieved using a steam distiller machine. It is simple; you fill the chamber of water, which is essentially a large electric kettle. You press the on button and the chamber heats the water to a boil. The boiling water becomes a sterilized steam vapor, which separates itself from all the contaminants below. The steam is directed into a condenser where the molecules cool and turn back into its liquid form, dripping down into the exit nozzle where it passes a final carbon filter pod to remove any potential VOCs (volatile organic compounds) that occasionally get sucked up with the vapor. These VOCs have a lower boiling point than water. Still, it is nothing to worry about as most distiller machines have this activated carbon pod, which is very efficient at making sure VOCs do not make it to the final water container. After leaving the carbon pod, the water collects into a glass container that is now ready to be used. Pure water the way nature intended it to be. There is absolutely no better way.

You will not have to shell out a fortune to buy a good distiller. You can get some for as cheap as around $50, though I recommend going with a higher-priced stainless steel distiller from a reputable company. You will most likely be using it a lot, so you want a reliable product. You can get distillers of all sizes, some top-loading where you manually load in the water. Other types are automatic and usually able to process much larger volumes throughout the day. You will need to research which styles are best for your budget, the space you have available, and how much time you want to spend loading the water.

I am happy with my current water setup, though I have dreams of one day having a system to automatically distribute distilled water throughout the whole house, including the shower! I use a 5-stage R.O. filter by APEC as the pre-filter. This unit is below the sink and it automatically fills a tank, so it is always full. I take that R.O. water and manually load a gallon into my countertop distiller, which produces a gallon of steam-distilled water in about 5 hours. I have a stainless steel distiller made by H2OLabs. I take that freshly distilled water and pour it into a three-gallon reservoir tank with a nozzle from which I dispense the water for drinking and cooking. On average, I would make about three gallons of distilled water per day for two people. I could distill the tap water directly, but using the R.O. water helps remove the debris that would build up in the distiller, which means I do not have to clean it as often. It is quite eye-opening to see the mysterious yellow slimy gunk that the water vapor leaves behind. That is a condensed conglomeration of what we put into our bodies when we drink tap water. Steam distillation is nature's perfect filter. Rather than additives like the governments use, or separating the toxins from the water like most filters, this process extracts the water from the toxins. Again, there is absolutely no better way to produce pure, drinkable water.

The next stage of my water research has led to investigating what is known as structured water. I have not had a chance to implement this yet, though I believe it will be the next level of my pure water system. There are four phases of water, and it has to do with the way water molecules position themselves in certain situations. Water has stimulating properties when put under different experiences. If you want an eye-opening discovery, look into reading the book by Masaru Emoto called *The Hidden Messages In Water*. This Japanese scientist discovered that water crystals could form elaborate shapes relating to the observer's consciousness or thoughts. Emoto shows real photographs of these shapes acting out the observer's emotions, which is implied by a written word or cadence of music. The most beautiful crystal is this magnificent hexagonal, multi-layered crystal formed by the words "Love and Gratitude." Other more hostile words such as "I Hate You" produced distorted, off-color blobs. It is almost as if the water could create conscious formations out of previous memory using thoughts as the blueprint. These photographs bridged the gap in metaphysical (consciousness) science to the physical realm, with water as the conduit between these dimensions. Spiritual to physical, all in the visual evidence of a photograph. Consciousness certainly is linked to water. I believe it is safe to assume that if we strive for higher vibrations of thought and emotion, then perfectly pure water will only further that pursuit.

QUOTES ON PURE WATER

I would like to point out this water knowledge is not of my own mind or just a few others. There are plenty of genius people throughout history who share the same sentiment on distilled water being the only pure water that humans should be drinking. I have compiled a small list of quotes from some people that you may know to hear what others are saying.

"I have KEPT UP MY DRINKING OF DISTILLED WATER and I attribute

my almost perfect health largely to it." — Dr. Alexander Graham Bell, Inventor of the Telephone

"To the best of our knowledge, there would not be any adverse health effects from THE CONTINUED INGESTION OF DISTILLED WATER." — Jack A. Bell – Assistant Director, May 17 1985; American Medical Association; Division of Personal and Public Health Policy

"Distilled Water is a pure water. A lot of people have been misled into believing that it robs minerals out of the body. Well, in my life, I've been DRINKING DISTILLED WATER FOR 35 YEARS. University of California Los Angeles, several years ago, told me I had the bone density of a 22-year-old athlete. So, if in fact Distilled Water robbed the body of minerals, I would probably be crippled by now" — Dr. Brian Clement, from the video, "Why Choose Distilled Water?"

"I personally have been DRINKING A GALLON OF DISTILLED WATER PER DAY for over 40 years. I fast all food for a minimum of 21 days annually. Over the years I have done three 40-day fasts on just distilled water. I fasted a year ago for 60 days: 40 days, then a break of 6 days eating only vegetables, and then continued another 20 days (for a total of 60 out of 66 days). No "early death" here, just perfect health and longevity." — Douglas Hoover, author of "Distilled Water and Health," Founder of Aquamedia Research Group, DistilledWaterAuthourity.com and DistillationStation.com

"If one plunges a watertight vessel of wax into the ocean, it will hold, after 24 hours, a certain quantity of water, that filtered into it through the waxen walls, and THIS WATER WILL BE FOUND TO BE POTABLE, BECAUSE THE EARTHY AND SALTY COMPONENTS HAVE BEEN SIEVED OFF." — Aristotle, from Meterologica (II. 3), First

published in 350 BC.

"While the two methods described above will kill most microbes in water, DISTILLATION WILL REMOVE MICROBES (GERMS) THAT RESIST THESE METHODS, as well as heavy metals, salts, and most other chemicals. Distillation involves boiling water and then collecting only the vapor that condenses. THE CONDENSED VAPOR WILL NOT INCLUDE SALT OR MOST OTHER IMPURITIES" — American Red Cross

10

PARASITES

A silent epidemic we are facing is the rise of parasitic infestation. It is a common myth in developed countries that only those who have traveled to a third-world country or ingested a Mexican tapeworm as a weight-loss strategy are the only ones who are at risk of hosting parasites. The reality is staunchly opposite of that. We come in contact with parasites in our food and water supply regularly. The eggs of most parasite species are microscopic and transferred in many different ways, such as through the air, on doorknobs, shaking hands, toilet seats, and sexual contact. The statistics are very hard to track as many people do not know about their parasites; however, the World Health Organization estimates that over 85% of the North American population is carrying at least one kind of parasite.

The word for parasite originates from the Greek meaning "one who eats off the table of another." These uninvited visitors can be microscopic such as fungus, yeast, or Protozoa, a single-celled organism that can invade any of the cells throughout your body. They can travel through the bloodstream and tissue,

84

much like the Lyme bacteria. The parasites can also be large and visible without a microscope. These larger body feeders are usually worms such as tapeworms, roundworms, and pinworms, among many others. These larger uninvited guests typically like to live in the digestive tract like the intestines, as this is where all the broken-down food particles are, which makes it very easy to leech. These worms can lay thousands of eggs per day in your system and reproduce the colony population quickly if not controlled.

It is unfortunate that even if you are reading this and want to know if you have any squatters taking up residence in your body, there is really no way to know what is living inside you. There are thousands of different species that can live in humans, and we only have tests for less than a hundred; the rest go undetected. Most of these infectious critters can live for decades without you having much evidence that you are infected. They know that if your body dies, they die with it, so they keep it alive just enough for you to function and continue to feed them. Even though they may not cause any directly debilitating symptoms, they cause underlying systemic issues for your body that worsen as the parasite colonies grow in both populations and physical size. Researchers are starting to see correlations with parasite infections and diseases such as heart disease, arthritis, asthma, diabetes, and cancer, though this needs to be studied further to make any relatable claims. Whether they cause those types of diseases or not, they surely do not help your body's immune system fight them off. That is why immune system dysfunction, like that created by Lyme disease, is an open invitation to intruders.

Each of the different parasite species can infect different parts of your body, usually the vital organs. For example, round-worms, also known as Ascaris, often infiltrate the lungs causing bronchial disorders. Hookworms latch on to the intestine walls and feed on the blood vessels, which can provoke numerous problems such as anemia. Fluke worms seem to favor the pancreas. Pinworms thrive around the reproductive and sexual organs. This list could continue, but I hope you see the urgency here; these organisms can be widespread inside your body, causing all sorts of systemic health problems. Also important to understand is these multi-celled organisms can host bacteria such as Lyme spirochetes, fungi, mold, and the like. Frequently people will be treated for Lyme disease, but it only takes them so far before they hit the ceiling with their recovery. This incomplete recovery could be due to the parasitic infection that is transporting and protecting the Lyme bacteria, not to mention creating other health problems. The worm species mainly cause a considerable health impact as they act as a sponge for heavy metals that the body is trying to eliminate. Not only are they trapping toxic waste like metals and bacteria in the body but also creating their own waste and leeching the beneficial vitamins and essential minerals. All of this is extremely taxing for our systems. That is the reason to fight off the parasites, and you would strongly benefit from an overall detox of your body's systems. Thankfully there are plenty of natural herbs that do a great job with fighting off the intruders, elimination of waste, and detoxification.

Before the 19th century, it was a common practice to de-worm yourself periodically. Being proactive with a parasite cleanse every six months is much more useful than waiting years until you potentially house a mass infestation. It is much easier to rid yourself of smaller younger parasites than trying to kill off a thirty-foot-long tapeworm! That being said, I understand that if you are reading this, you are probably just realizing the parasite problem. Let's move forward and discuss some ways you can remove parasites from your body.

I did not expect I would have any serious parasites in my body. Sure, maybe fungus on my toenails or some yeast built up, but aside from the Lyme, I thought there was nothing else afflicting my body. After researching this topic, I decided to try a parasite cleanse protocol. I had nothing to lose, and after all, I was using natural substances that are safe for your body regardless of pests residing or not. I was astounded, shocked, and horrified after a few weeks of the cleanse when I passed what looked like a tapeworm about ten inches in length! I thought, how could I possibly have worms?! I know I have been in Africa and Thailand, but I only ate from quality sources. I learned that it did not matter; quality sources or not, I had worms. And it probably had nothing to do with my travels. Weeks went on as I continued to pass roundworms up to twelve inches or longer. Each elimination of a new parasite was creepy, yet I was relieved that my cleanse was working. Seeing these entities removed from inside my body with my own eyes was a real psychological challenge. I suddenly became utterly disgusted with the human body and wanted nothing to do with it. I was no longer attracted to anyone, and the thought of any physical interaction with other people repulsed me. That was a huge problem that leached into my personal life, which caused obstacles in the relationship with my long-term girlfriend. We became physically and emotionally disconnected due to the war going on inside my mind. I had to get over this psychological block that I now had about the human body. I needed time. It seemed I had to focus first on eliminating the parasites, and then I could start rebuilding my mindset.

DIATOMACEOUS EARTH

First, I learned about Diatomaceous Earth (DE) and its effectiveness in killing off intruders in the digestive tract. That was the first substance I began taking, which led to the passing of that first giant worm. DE is a safe and effective way to start clearing out your system. This white powdery substance is fossilized algae. It is made of ancient hexagon-shaped organisms with silicon exoskeletons called diatoms that are ground up and ready for ingestion. Many people may have heard of using this for dogs or other house pets, but when you use the food-grade quality, it is safe and effective for human consumption. Another benefit to ingesting this substance is that it is high in vitamins and nutrients that you may not be getting elsewhere; one example is silica, which helps strengthen the connective tissues in the brain and spinal cord. It also helps build healthy hair, skin, and nails.

Diatomaceous Earth is effective at removing both the tiny and the more substantial invaders. It traps the microscopic parasites along with heavy metal particles and carries them out of your body. For the bigger worms, the particles sweep through and slice the worms to bits over time. It will kill off the bigger parasites, and your intestines will naturally flush them out through regular elimination. That sounds harsh; however, DE cannot cut through your intestinal lining, making it a very gentle and safe way to treat an infestation. You will want to take one tablespoon of DE mixed in water or a smoothie twice a day for a few weeks or even months before moving on to the next protocol substance.

MIMOSA PUDICA

After a few months of taking Diatomaceous Earth, I had only passed one parasite that looked to be segmented exactly like a tapeworm. I wondered if that was the only thing living in me and if I had eliminated the problem; however, I intuitively felt there was more to be removed. I continued taking DE and added the next and most effective substance to my treatment: Mimosa Pudica (MP). You may have seen this plant out in nature as it has an exciting mechanism that attracts attention. It is known as the Sensitive Plant because of its defensive mechanism that is triggered when being touched. You can touch the tiny symmetrical leaves and they will start moving and close up.

I learned about Mimosa Pudica through Dr. Jay Davidson's book *How To Fix Lyme Disease*. Dr. Davidson mentions how he passed a few very large worms after taking this substance while battling Lyme, so I figured I might as well give it a try, especially after seeing one worm eliminated, which is clear evidence that there are more that need to pass. After some research, it was clear that the MP seeds are the most potent part of the plant. The seed works like a sticky intestinal scrubber that sweeps through and picks up debris, including parasites, toxins, immobile food waste, etc. It becomes the street sweeper of your digestive tract. I made sure to purchase a supplement that was all seed. I began taking capsules from a company called Microbe Formulas, the same brand mentioned in that book. It is a fantastic product as it is 100% MP seed in the capsule. I would take two capsules in the morning and two at night, paired with another product from the same company called BioTox, which is activated carbon to help bind and flush the waste out of my body. Immediately these two substances worked very well together! Within just a few days, I began seeing results in almost every elimination that lasted for over a month. To my surprise, I passed a couple of roundworms even larger than before. I began to feel relief in my abdominal area that I had not expected. I wondered how long I must have been hoarding these pesky invaders, but I did not care, I was just ecstatic to see them go!

If you decide to try a parasite protocol, keep in mind that statistically, less than 30% of parasites found in the human body are visible. If you do not see anything obvious in your stool that does not mean that it is not working, you could not have any large multi-celled organisms in your body. Usually, a parasite cleansing protocol should be daily and consistent for at least four months. It also helps to switch up protocol methods. If you start taking DE for a few months, try abruptly changing it up to MP and BioTox for the next couple of months. Actually, since MP is also a binder, you could continue taking that while introducing a new combative substance. Some other substances that are effective at killing parasites are vidanga, neem, wormwood, black walnut, and clove. You may find it practical to introduce some of those substances after going through the previously mentioned protocols.

A word of caution: attacking parasites is very similar to attacking Lyme. The higher doses you take, the more waste your body will need to get rid of in a short amount of time. Once again, this is known as the Herxheimer reaction. If you cannot tolerate the extreme brain fog or achy pains that may come with treatment, then it is recommended you start slowly and work your way up. Two capsules of MP twice daily is a low dose, you could ramp that up to six capsules twice daily if you want to conduct an all-out attack on the invaders. You will be safe taking large natural substances, just pay attention to your body and know your physical, mental, and emotional limits. This approach is a long-term play; if the parasites have been accumulating for years, you will not get rid of them overnight. It may take six months to a year or longer to see the elimination taper off. The good news is that you should start to feel better before then!

After all of this repulsive parasite elimination, it was time to rebuild my mindset. I have accepted the parasite reality instead of resisting it. It has helped me to come to terms with the fact that my body is not always my own and that I share it with many different life forms. I focus on eating the best natural foods as possible and avoiding low-quality food sources. Most worms are found in meats and fish, so thankfully, I am already avoiding those risk factors because of the Lyme. A few weeks ago, my friend sent me a picture of her fish she bought at Costco with a four-inch worm right there in the fish's flesh. It does not matter where you live; these worms and other parasites are everywhere. The good news is now you know, and being aware of the issue, you can make smarter choices.

The first step is to eliminate what may be in your body already through the protocols above and any other methods you find useful. While combating your parasites, you can learn how to reduce or remove exposure to new critters by eating clean, avoiding meat and dairy, avoiding processed foods, and avoid buying groceries from disreputable markets. Once you have that figured out and you have successfully eliminated the majority of your intruders, maintain an annual or biannual protocol for keeping any new parasite colonies from growing. This may sound daunting, but this just takes a little change upfront, and then you can put all of this on autopilot so that you can optimize your life. That is what this is all about! Once all of this was on autopilot, I was able to love myself and be okay with residing in my physical form. Since I was now able to love myself, it was easier to find an attraction for the human body again. Through meditation, yoga, self-development, and soul growth practices, I could evolve my mind and my heart beyond the consciousness of my former self that began this journey. This adversity will surely strengthen your resolve. Push forward. Everyone has the right to overcome these challenges; believe that for yourself, take action, and you will get through to the other side.

11

ELECTROMAGNETIC RADIATION

"If you want to find the secrets of the universe, think in terms of energy, frequency, and vibration." – Nikola Tesla

Biologically speaking, anyone that has a weakened immune system or is fighting off illness is more at risk of becoming ill with other afflictions. Your autoimmune response can only handle so much before it is overworked and outnumbered. As I am writing this, the Coronavirus is sweeping through the entire planet. I am sure you have heard to stay away from the elderly as they have weaker immune systems, which means they will easily pick up the virus and not be able to defend against it, which puts them in a fatal risk. Those of us with Lyme are in a similar position. Until we defeat the Lyme bacteria and rebuild the immune system, we are temporarily weaker and more at risk of attracting other illnesses. It is clear that in the event of battling through Lyme disease (or any other disease), we should do everything possible to eliminate those risk factors that may be weakening our recovery.

In the circumstance of battling Lyme disease, many environmental factors can play a role in how fast or slow you can heal. You may know stories of workplace environmental toxicities discovered years after they have caused people severe health problems. For example, asbestos used in the walls of buildings finally proved to cause lung cancer. For decades this substance surrounded people without anyone realizing the harm it was doing to their health. It took many decades to validate the research and then begin the expensive removal of the toxic materials from their surroundings. There is a new dangerous toxin penetrating the fabric of our society. It is between the walls of our workplace, the halls of our children's schools, the hospital rooms of our sick, the nursing homes of our elderly, the living rooms of our homes. It is even in the outside open-air spaces of our cities; this new wave of toxicity is called electromagnetic radiation.

Electromagnetic radiation (EMR) is also known as electromagnetic frequencies. If you are not sure what this is yet, let me use some words to help you understand: WIFI, hotspot, Bluetooth, cell phone reception or signal, 3G, 4G, 5G, 6G, etc. Our society has become so inundated with technology that the digital world has almost overtaken the real natural world for a lot of people. If you live in a developed area, chances are you cannot go to many places without being surrounded by electrical power lines, TV screens, digital billboards, smart appliances, and mobile devices like your cell phone and laptop computer. Electromagnetic radiation is like the modern-day asbestos problem; only it is a silent and invisible weapon that is far more prevalent, popping up in more and more locations each day. It is bombarding our bodies every second of the day that we are among civilization.

If legislators do not soon recognize the research showing how harmful these frequencies are, we will be a very sick society. EMR is, in itself, a global pandemic problem.

HEALTH CONCERNS

It is essential to understand that in nature, there exist many frequencies. Everything that exists in life has a frequency vibrating at specific rates. For example, a sound wave vibrating at a low rate will produce a low sound. As it increases in rate, the sound pitch will get higher. With physical matter, it works the same way; different elements or materials will vibrate at different frequency rates. Inside the human body are cells that operate on their own natural frequencies. Frequencies are states of information. There are healing frequencies, and there are harmful ones. Our cells transmit their biological information throughout the body, and this messaging system gets convoluted when exposed to external frequency information. A scientist from Eastern State University named Bruce Tainio developed a frequency monitor in which he could measure the frequency outputs of the human body. His discovery shows the human body has a rate of 62 to 68 Hertz (Hz). He then discovered when the frequency dropped below that threshold to 52 Hz it would develop flu-like symptoms. Even further down to 42 Hz and below would easily develop cancer. That is very important to understand; different frequencies will create different matter. When our cell vibrations are disturbed by other permeating frequencies, they start to break down and malfunction. On an energetic level, this creates a perfect storm of biological problems.

The Swedish National Institute for Working Life performed a study in 2006 which found that people who used cell phones for over two thousand hours (accumulating over time) had a 240 percent or higher risk of developing a malignant tumor on the side of their head that the phone is held against. That is just one of the many health issues that cell phones can create. Other health problems caused by cell phone radiation include emotional and behavioral disorders in children, leukemia, hormone disruption, sleep disorders, immune-system suppression, depression, brain fog, memory problems, headaches, chronic fatigue syndrome, fibromyalgia, DNA damage, anxiety, heart arrhythmias, arthritis, breathing and asthma problems, infertility, and so many more disorders. This list could go on and on. Many doctors and health care professionals are talking about how, in the last two decades, there has been a sharp rise in mystery illnesses and symptoms. These mysterious symptoms are not obviously traced back to any studied illness or disease they learned about in medical school. It is as if all of a sudden, the human body just started acting haywire for no detectable reason. It makes sense that an untraceable source is causing these untraceable symptoms.

Many experts have seen a link between these mysterious symptoms of chronic illness and the increase of EMR exposure. We now live in a society saturated in these harmful frequencies. This radiation bath is no help to those battling Lyme disease. Lyme disease has been around for a long time now, and one cannot help but wonder why the number of cases seems to be exponentially on the rise? Is it Lyme awareness? Maybe. Are there higher quantities of ticks? Probably. Have the ticks been manipulated and weaponized by the government (read the book

Bitten by Kris Newby)? The answer is actually yes to all of these questions, but also it is very plausible that Lyme disease was not as debilitating before EMR exposure. Research shows that Lyme symptoms are more manageable to deal with or to recover from without constant EMR exposure. Dr. Dietrich Klinghardt had more success treating Lyme with EMR shielding than he did with using antibiotics. His research led him to the conclusion that the EMR waves drive the microbes to become more aggressive inside the body. The key for Lyme recovery is to eliminate exposure to all other toxicities while treating the Lyme. If you can treat the Lyme while removing yourself from most environmental toxins such as EMR, mold, heavy metal intake, dead foods, impure water, stress, corrupt media, negative thought patterns, and other parasites, you should find yourself on a fast-track to optimal health, free of Lyme symptoms.

EMR is not only dangerous to those of us with Lyme disease but instead to all living forms. Humans, animals, plants, and insects are all biology that is affected by these harmful waves. Our most common exposure is usually due to the mobile phone and cellular towers. Almost everyone in the developing world carries one on them at nearly every hour of the day. A study published in 2013 stated that EMR has a non-thermal chemical impact on human cells. The frequencies can drive calcium out of their cells and damage the potassium ions, which help control brain function. Lithium in the brain is also affected by EMR disturbing mental stability. Think about that the next time you take a phone call and put the device right up against your skull. A British scientist named Andrew Goldsworthy, Ph.D. has a theory that since one in four car accidents is due to a driver on a phone call, the reason is not that the driver is distracted by the call but rather the brain function is distorted and slowed by the EMR waves permeating the brain cells, flooding them with calcium ions (calcium atoms electrically charged). This hypothesis checks out when you compare it to similar cases of human function disrupted around high doses of EMR. One study of young adults in Australia found a link to high cell phone usage and poor cognitive function with delayed reaction times.

WHY IS THIS LEGAL?

Many countries around the world are acknowledging the damage EMR can do to their citizens. Belgium recently banned mobile phone use for children under the age of seven years old. Belgium's capital city Brussels was also the first to ban 5G wireless due to health concerns. 5G is supposed to be far more deadly than the current wireless networks. Thankfully these types of bans and resistance to the 5G network are accumulating more and more support. In 2017, a large group of scientists and doctors from all around the world sent an appeal to the European Union over the extreme dangers of 5G and to halt building 5G infrastructure. To quote a paragraph from the top of the paper: *"We the undersigned, more than 180 scientists and doctors from 36 countries, recommend a moratorium on the roll-out of the fifth generation, 5G, for telecommunication until potential hazards for human health and the environment have been fully investigated by scientists independent from industry. 5G will substantially increase exposure to radiofrequency electromagnetic fields (RF-EMF) on top of the 2G, 3G, 4G, Wi-Fi, etc. for telecommunications already in place. RF-EMF has been proven to be harmful for humans and the environment."* One of the leaders in this initiative is Dr. L. Hardell, Professor of Oncology at Örebro University which is in

Sweden. His message is clear: *"The telecom industry is trying to roll out technology that may have very real, unintended harmful consequences. Scientific studies, both recently and over many years, have identified harmful effects on health when testing wireless products under realistic conditions. We are very concerned that the increase in radiation exposure by 5G leads to damage that cannot be reversed".*

Hardell also states: *"The fifth generation (5G) of radio frequency radiation is now being developed. This is done without dosimetric determination or study of the possible health effects. The media praise in particular all the possibilities that this technology promises to offer, such as the self-propelled car and Internet of Things (IoT). The consequences for the health of humans, plants and animals are not discussed at all. Politicians, governments and the media are responsible for unbalanced information. Ordinary people are not informed of conflicting opinions about this technological development. Health effects from radio frequency radiation are a non issue in the media, at least in Sweden, but also in most other countries".*

Slowly the countries of the world are waking up. The United States will most likely be one of the last countries to recognize health concerns, especially if reducing or eliminating the problem will threaten the profits of mega-corporations who control the industry. Unfortunately, the U.S. legislation is for sale by high-power lobbyist groups and backroom deals for the politicians. Over the last few decades, there has been a corporate take-over of the political system. No longer are the days that laws and regulations are put in place for the citizens' safety and well-being. Those days have long gone; now, laws are written to accommodate the wishes of the highest bidder. To quote an article from the Scientific American publication in 2006: *"Also it is important to remember that, perhaps expectedly, interpretations of findings in this area of investigations are shrouded in controversy, particularly because special interests may influence some of the research."* To state more clearly, once again, the companies that profit from the telecommunication frequencies are the same groups controlling the safety research.

In February 2010, GQ Magazine put out an article confirming that corporations do not care for the well-being of the people: *"The Telecommunications Act of 1996 - a watershed for the cell phone industry - was the result, in part, of nearly fifty million dollars in political contributions and lobbying largesse from the telecom industry. The prize in the TCA for telecom companies branching into wireless was a rider known as Section 704, which specifically prohibits citizens and local governments from stopping placement of a cell tower due to health concerns. Section 704 was clear: There could be no litigation to oppose cell towers because the signals make you sick."* That is one of many articles displaying the corruption and for-profit-negligence in the legislative and corporate clubhouse. The government is for sale to the corporations, and the corporations do not care about your health. We can only hope the rest of the world continues on with the awareness and prevention of 5G and other dangerous frequencies until the U.S. is peer pressured into following suit.

**Special word of hope: As of January 2020, new evidence has come into view that the 5G grid in the United States may have upgraded to remove the dangers from the frequency output. The towers may have upgraded with a magnetic alloy with an extremely high flux* *density Cobalt (Co-49%), Iron (Fe-49%), and Vanadium (V-2%). The magnets have been shown to clean up the impurities from 5G on an ionic level. This would prevent oxygen from being depleted, which would render the 5G frequencies harmless. We will have to watch as more information is released.*

HOW TO REDUCE EXPOSURE

It may seem overwhelming to begin the process of reducing your EMR exposure in a world saturated in frequencies. Take a look around your home, and you will probably see dozens of electronic devices all outputting harmful waves. The dangers are not just in the communication devices, but any equipment or infrastructure that uses electricity. All electric devices put out at least a low electromagnetic field (ELF). These are less dangerous than the radio communications but are usually the frequencies that are continually exposing us (for example, if you live under power lines). So to not get overwhelmed with all of this, I have found it most comfortable to start by removing or reducing the most significant EMR contributors. In other words, control that which you can manage and try not to worry about the problems outside of your control. Below is the list of your most-likely daily threats of EMR exposure.

Cell phones and cordless phones: Whatever you do, keep your mobile device away from your body as much as possible! I have tested my cell phone with a radio frequency meter to measure the exposure and it was over 1000 times more than the recommended safety limit! Imagine what this can do over the years of usage. You can get wired headphones for phone calls and hold it out away from your head. If that is not possible, then at least put the phone on speaker and hold it away from your body. Remember, studies show the more prolonged and closer the device is to your skull, the more prone to developing a tumor on that side of your head. When you sleep at night you should have your phone on airplane mode or turn it off completely. I am not a parent so my parenting advice is not valid. However, this health advice is validated by research; if you are a new parent, you indeed should not be scrolling aimlessly on social media with the phone next to your newborn baby's head (I see this situation very frequently). That should also be a guide for positioning baby monitors as well. Avoid carrying your phone in your pants pocket next to your reproductive organs, as this may contribute to our society's rise of infertility problems. You may be able to find a phone case that reduces the EMR though this can only do so much. All in all, limit usage time as much as possible and stay as far away as you can from your device until you need it.

WI-FI: Like all EMR, the Wi-Fi is proximity-based. That means the closer you are to the router, the more dangerous it will be for you. It would be wise to position your Wi-Fi router in a room that you are rarely in, like a basement or a spare room. The worst place to put your router is your bedroom or any child's bedroom. It helps to set the router in an area that can be easily unplugged or switched off at night while you sleep. That way, you don't have harmful waves seeping into your body while trying to rest and repair itself overnight. The best-case scenario is having your internet connection hardwired, though I know it is a challenge with all the portable smart devices we rely on now. Make sure you do not sit near the routers at work or school since these are usually much stronger of a signal. If you are near these devices, it is okay to address your concerns and request to move elsewhere.

Along with the harmful connective waves, the devices themselves also output ELFs. Staring at a computer or phone screen for hours each day can damage the eyes. Having a laptop or tablet on your lap can create harm to your cells. It helps to be mindful of how close your electronics are to your biology and operate accordingly. Cell phones, computers, and Wi-Fi have become a necessity in our way of life, but if you can be conscious enough to reduce your exposure, you will prevent or at least reduce the adverse health effects.

Bluetooth: The same rules that apply to cell phones and Wi-Fi routers apply to Bluetooth devices. Stay as far away from the gadget as possible and reduce exposure as much as you can. Thankfully Bluetooth waves are much weaker and do not expand out too far, especially through the walls. The real dangerous situation I see is the latest technology trend of wireless earbuds. It seems to be a wonderfully convenient gadget; no cords are hanging from your ears! The problem is that you have two devices receiving dangerous frequencies directly next to your brain. I am appalled when I see young children wearing these devices. Their developing brains are far more susceptible to EMR damage. The recommendation for these devices is to strictly never use them. Do not put them anywhere near your head, especially for long durations of time like a gym workout or lengthy phone call. Revert back to wired headphones, ideally ones made for low EMR exposure with air tube wires where the electricity is not flowing alongside your head.

Microwave: The microwave is one of the most convenient

kitchen appliances, especially if you eat a lot of prepared pack-aged foods. Most often, a product's main instructions for heating the dish involves the microwave. What you have not learned in these instructions is that the microwave will destroy any micronutrients left in the food. All the vitamins and essential minerals that your dish may have contained rupture by the time the food is hot. It has reduced to lifeless matter. You are better off not eating at all than eating the damaged microwaved food. Not only is the microwave killing your food nutrition, but the waves are also leaking out of the door and into the kitchen. These devices are designed to meet government standards on leakage, and according to radiation expert Larry Gust, these standards are thousands of times higher than they should be for safe use. The radiation leaks right through the microwave window into whoever is standing nearby. Many new kitchens now have the microwave up above the stove at eye level, which is the worst place for the microwave. You do not want this device anywhere near your body and especially not your head. The good news is it does not take that much more time to put the food contents into a pot and heat it the natural way over a stovetop. I encourage you to try heating food up without the microwave for a while, and you will see it is not that much more work. And besides, even if it is more work, your health and family's health is worth the extra few minutes of labor.

Smart Meters: Throughout many of the developed countries, the power companies are going around to every home and installing new smart meter devices. They will tell you it helps them gauge the usage better to save you money, which sounds good, but what they do not tell you is the dangers of these devices. The first danger, smart meters are a fire hazard. There have been hundreds of cases of house fires that were traced back to the smart meter shorting out and causing an electrical fire. The second danger of these smart meters is the radiation output. Many people have experienced feeling sick or even chronic illness from prolonged exposure to their smart meters. And unfortunately, you cannot do much to avoid exposure to these devices like you can to a cell phone. The smart meters are installed in a fixed location on your house, sometimes directly outside a bedroom wall just a foot from where a person sleeps! It becomes especially dangerous in apartment complexes when someone may be living on the other side of a wall with dozens of meters, each outputting harmful radiation waves.

In an article written by Michele Hertz, founder of Stop Smart Meters NY, the problem is clearly stated: *"Electronic meters contain fragile miniaturized electronic circuit boards that are prone to igniting and exploding when exposed to utility-side electrical fire risk events and outdoor weather conditions. These meters pose unacceptable hazards because they lack essential electrical safety components -circuit breakers and surge arrestors. The installation of electronic meters on homes and businesses has resulted in hundreds of thousands of reported health, fire, electrical, privacy, and overbilling complaints and incidents. According to cyber-security experts, electronic meters are an unaddressed and looming threat to the utility grid and public safety. Many thousands of these meters have been recalled. By contrast, mechanical analog utility meters have been in place in the United States for decades. They have been the subject of few, if any, reported complaints or unsafe incidents. Analog meters are electrical and contain no ignitable or energy consuming electronic components. Analog meters protect privacy and pose no cyber-security breach risks. Analog meters have no history of being recalled."*

Depending on what state you live in, you may be able to opt-out of the smart meter installation. Each state is different, so you will have to do some research on what you can do to protect your household. Fight as hard and as long as you can to keep your analog meter in place. The government needs to know the people are not going to submit to the power companies when the health of our families is at risk. We do not want these harmful, privacy-encroaching devices in our homes. Do what you can, research as much as possible, and fight to have this smart meter removed or blocked from being installed.

X-Rays: I once assumed that because hospitals and doctor offices use X-ray machines that they are safe. I was incorrect in that assumption. X-ray machines are hazardous and should only be used if absolutely necessary. The way dentists and doctors haphazardly recommend x-rays seems counterintuitive. The World Health Organization, the Center for Disease Control and Prevention, and the National Institute of Environmental Health Sciences all classify x-rays as a carcinogen. They say frequent x-rays at high doses can cause an assortment of different cancers. The New England Journal of Medicine published a study that showed one in fifty cancers were caused by imaging machines such as x-ray, MRI, or CT scans. That means that if you are going for a mammogram to make sure you don't have cancer in your breast, over time your chances are high that those breast scans actually give you what you are hoping not to find! It is a backward system, indeed.

I had a dentist growing up that insisted on conducting an x-ray on my mouth every single time I went for a cleaning. I visited his office three to four times per year. That is a lot of radiation exposure for a young boy. Now, as an adult, I understand why he pushed for frequent imaging. When the doctor or dentist owns their own machine, they want to use it to pay for itself and bring in more profit. They can easily use their authority as a doctor to self-refer patients to get an x-ray on their machine. This expense is then billed back to the insurance company (if they have insurance), and the doctor makes more revenue with each x-ray. The Washington Post did an investigation in this matter and found that within a few months of one Midwest doctor purchasing a CT scanner, the number of scans suggested rose by 700%. Now obviously, not every doctor or dentist will do this just for money. However, it is something to be aware of; it does happen quite often. If you are told that you need imaging done, think through any other prevention methods or diagnostic options before jumping into the radiation methods. Of course, there are many times these imaging machines have saved people's lives by finding something, but they have also caused harm to people. This subtle warning is just to make you aware there may be another safer way to maintain your health and make sure it is necessary before going through with any scans.

12

MAINTENANCE

When the dream is big enough, the obstacles don't matter.

I intend that by the time you get to this chapter, you have already taken action on a few of the treatment methods mentioned in previous chapters. Ideally, you are already feeling some symptoms letting up or have hope that you will soon. Or maybe you just started and are bogged down from the Herxheimer reaction; that is okay too. Just keep pushing forward with your treatments. It may take weeks or months to feel any sense of physical or mental relief from the symptoms. There is a world of optimal health waiting for you, and I believe anyone with Lyme disease, no matter how debilitating it is, can come back to good health. Once you defeat the Lyme battle, which you will, you will need to know how to maintain your good health over time. If you stop these treatments as soon as you feel great again and go back to your previous way of life, the chances are very high that you will slowly regain your Lyme disease symptoms. I know you do not want to be pulled back down into that dark place again. Thankfully, once you return to good health, it is easy to stay there with some small, conscious, and consistent efforts.

Diet: The food you eat from this time forward is probably the most critical symptom prevention method. It will be tempting to go back to your old favorite foods, but I encourage you to stick with your new healthier diet. For me, I still get tempted by doughnuts. Gluten and sugar-heavy foods always capture my cravings. I occasionally cave to the desires and usually regret it; however, I am okay with it now and then. Of course, it is up to you if you want to try to test your body and see how it reacts to food now, but often Lyme disease has changed your body permanently. In cases where Lyme caused an allergy to red meat or gluten, it will most likely remain that way even after you rid yourself of Lyme symptoms. It helps to think of your battle with Lyme disease as the wake-up call you needed to start living a healthier lifestyle. There are plenty of ways to enjoy food more healthily, so find what foods work for you and I encourage you to stick with it!

Samento and Banderol: It would be wise to keep these two battle-tested warriors on call. I usually keep a 2 oz bottle of both Samento and Banderol in my supplements cabinet so that they are readily available when needed. I would recommend circling back to go through these bottles every six months for a few years. Doing this will make sure any lingering Lyme bacteria hiding out will not have a chance to make a comeback. You may need to continue some of these protocols for as long as you live, a small price for a great result. Once again, this protocol is very affordable, so it should not affect your finances too much and certainly will not harm your health to take it periodically. At this point, you should be able to jump right into a full dose twice each day rather than working your way up the protocol drop by drop. If that is too hard on your body, you can begin the protocol from the beginning. The goal is to eventually drink around thirty drops of Samento and thirty drops of Banderol in the morning and then again at night. This routine is a perfect maintenance protocol. Once you finish the bottles, you should be feeling very clear and at ease knowing the Lyme is safely at bay. After a few years of this, you may explore doing the protocol every year or even every other year. The longer you have been living a clean lifestyle, the less frequent you will need to use these amazing herbs. These timelines are what have worked for me, but of course, not all bodies are the same. Listen to your body; it should tell you how frequently you will need to take these supplements.

Ozone and Silver: It would be beneficial to circle back to these protocols periodically. Ideally, you can create your own silver and generate your own ozone at home for long-term use. If that is not manageable, then schedule these treatments as often as you can without going broke. Both of these treatments are tremendous for generally maintaining good health.

Parasite Protocol: As mentioned earlier, before the 19th century, it was a common practice to de-worm yourself periodically. Being proactive with a parasite cleanse every six months is much more effective than waiting years until you have a potential mass infestation. It is much easier to rid yourself of small younger parasites than trying to kill off a thirty-foot-long tapeworm! What I have done is every six months (in between the Samento and Banderol protocol), I would take Diatomaceous Earth mixed in water, along with capsules of Mimosa Pudica, and BioTox twice a day until the bottles of the capsules ran out. That approach seemed to reduce the sluggish drag that any parasitic afflictions had on my body.

I will most likely continue this protocol periodically for as long as I live because parasites are a constant risk as long as we are ingesting food. Thankfully, like the Samento and Banderol, this maintenance is also very affordable and easy to do. Overall, it helps to be mindful of avoiding parasitic foods as much as possible while maintaining a consistent de-worming schedule. I encourage you to explore the different herbs that function as parasitic cleanses and experiment to find which ones are most effective for your particular situation. Remember, it can take at least a few months for the first treatment to see or feel any results of parasitic elimination.

Meditation: Consistent meditation has proven to boost your immune system. In the fast-paced society in which most of us live, anxiety and stress are at an all-time high. Stress is a huge risk factor for disease and illness. Unfortunately, our school systems do not teach how to manage stress. Meditation can produce beautiful results. If you clear out the stress that has accumulated over your lifetime, it can significantly help your bodily systems function much more effectively, especially the immune system. There are many different meditation styles, and that can be overwhelming to a new person of interest. I encourage you to research a style that seems to interest you and would best fit your life.

What has been working for me is an approach called Effortless Meditation. I attempt to do twenty minutes in the morning and twenty minutes in the evening, though anything is better than nothing if there is time for only a fraction of that. I find a quiet place to close my eyes and silently repeat a one-word mantra repeatedly in my mind. Thoughts will come and go, but as soon as I am aware I have drifted off into a thought loop, I simply return to repeating the mantra. This repetition will entrain the brain and allow you to dive deeper into the mind below the turbulent ocean of mental noise. It will allow your body to reach a deeper state of rest, sometimes reaching a more profound rest than sleep can obtain. In this restful state, the body can release stress and begin to rebuild.

After months of developing a meditation practice, I have experienced less anxiety, higher intuition, increased creativity, greater empathy, smoother decision-making, better breathing function, reduced anger, feelings of joy, and many other positive attributes. I encourage you to give it a try for a few weeks. It helps to go into a new practice with zero expectations of what you may have heard about meditation. Meditation can be different for everyone, so the only way to honestly know what it can do for you is to give it a consistent effort, effortlessly.

Cutting back: The above covers the additive methods of maintenance, but what about the toxins we should leave out? Throughout your recovery, you will find it significantly easier to progress if you avoid some of the most common and socially-accepted toxins. The first one on this list is cigarettes. Everyone knows the dangers of smoking, and it is obvious it will have a negative effect on your body. The same can be said for alcohol. Alcohol suppresses the immune system, and your weakened Lyme body would have a better chance to recover without the extra poison in its system. Your kidneys and liver will need to be at their best during the beginnings of your battle with Lyme disease. I did not drink any alcohol for a few years during my recovery and have only recently allowed myself to drink natural red wine periodically. If you are a nightlife kind of person, at first your friends may not understand why you are not drinking with them. I have found that people respect your decision when you tell them you have Lyme disease and are doing everything you can to heal. You will probably start to feel proud of your resolve. Once you get over the initial uncomfortable social change, you will be thankful you cut back; I can guarantee that. You probably never heard anyone say they wish they drank more, but you certainly hear the opposite!

Fasting: Another excellent way of eliminating the intake of toxins to boost your immune system is by fasting. Technically, most of the available food in our modern-day society is considered waste to the body. After its ingestion, the body processes the food, extracts what it can use, stores some of it for later, and then pushes the rest out through elimination. The body does not need the majority of the food that is eaten, not to mention all the chemicals and additives found in a lot of products. The abundance of food that developed nations have access to can promote overindulgence. That relentless digestive process requires a lot of energy. Think about this, how free would your system be if there was no food to process? What else could your body focus on doing instead? Your highly intelligent body will begin to send support to other processes, like strengthening the immune system to attack other diseases that have been evolving. A full restoration of health will begin. To put it simply, your body will start to heal in a way that it cannot do so while processing the nonstop barrage of food intake.

Fasting expert, Joel Fuhrman, M.D. has a terrific book on the subject called *"Fasting and Eating for Health."* In the first chapter, the doctor states, "Therapeutic fasting is not a mystical or magical cure. It works because the body has within it the capacity to heal when the obstacles to healing are removed. Health is the normal state. [...] Fasting stops the continual work of the digestive tract, whose activity can drain the body of energy and divert the healing process." While there are many different styles and methods of fasting (juice fasting for example), Dr. Fuhrman makes the case that water fasting is the most powerful way of fasting. He declares, "One cannot, however, achieve the powerful benefits of complete fasting if juices are part of the fast. 'Juice fasting' is not truly fasting; biochemically the body does not enter the 'protein-sparing' fasting state. In this state the body conserves its muscle reserves and fat is preferentially broken down. This does not occur with juice fasting. Juice fasting also does not have the powerful anti-inflammatory properties of the pure water fast that are essential for recovery in autoimmune illnesses."

There are so many incredible results from long-term water fasting, and it is quite a broad topic of research, too large to do a deep dive in this book. If you are interested in obtaining the blessings of fasting, I will encourage you to read Dr. Fuhrman's book. After the bulk of my Lyme treatments, I began with a simple three-day fast. I ate healthy small portions leading up to it the two days before and fasted from a Friday morning through the weekend. I ate nothing and only drank water, no other juices or supplements. I began introducing food back into my body on Monday morning. That gave me confidence that I could go longer. If you never stopped eating for more than a day in your life, it can be a bizarre and scary feeling not to eat at all. After these three days, I knew I could go longer. A few months later I planned a seven day fast. At the start, the goal is to eat healthy natural plant-based meals two or three days before a prolonged fast, then the day before only ingesting juices and fruits with lots of water. During the fast, you should strive to drink approximately a gallon of water a day while getting lots of rest. You do not want to be standing or walking around too much. Strive for as little physical activity as possible!

The first day was easy to get through with spikes of hunger throughout the day, which eventually subsided. The second day was reasonably similar to the first day in how I felt. Day three was much more challenging. The cravings started to attack my mind. I kept getting flashes of my favorite foods, mainly Thai drunken noodles, which is one of my favorite dishes. I was also experiencing headaches and shaky muscles throughout the day. I had to keep my vision fresh in my mind. It helps to dangle the reason why you are doing this in front of you at all times. The dream is more important than the process. The most challenging day was day four out of the seven. This day was the most physically challenging and mentally torturing. I had numerous physical maladies such as fatigue, headaches, weak muscles, joint pain, bright flashes in my sight, and a nagging cough that surfaced. I thought the cough was probably a dormant respiratory issue that my body was finally able to eradicate. Mentally I was consumed with cravings, negative self-talk, doubts, worries, and the like. I almost caved because the cravings were so bad. It seemed equivalent to a drug addict needing a fix. Once again, when the dream is big enough, the obstacles don't matter. Thankfully I stuck with it, I knew by this point that I could not eat the food I was craving anyway as it would be too dangerous; you have to ease back into feeding. I was happy day four was over.

Waking up on day five was relieving. The cravings had gone, no more headaches. I was starting to feel energy again, and most importantly, my mindset had cleared back to a positive, optimistic state. What is happening around this point of a fast is the body has switched into a metabolic state of ketosis, meaning it is producing ketones to use as energy rather than using carbs or glucose. After your body makes this switch, most people can start feeling energized again. Even though the body may be feeling energized at this point, you will still want to take it easy so you do not burn through it all. Days six and seven were both positive, and I could tell the fast was effectively healing my body. These last two days were comfortable and almost fun to experience. I would have kept the fast going had it not been for a day ahead that week that I had to be physically-abled. I broke my fast on the eighth day. I drank watermelon juice in the morning, and then I ate some pieces of watermelon shortly after. Through the remainder of the day, I consumed small portions of fruit and juices. The following day I continued the fruit and introduced small portions of carbs throughout the day.

My next fasting endeavor is to water fast for twenty-one days or longer. The longer you can do a pure water fast, the better. Now that does not mean to go out and fast for thirty days without doing any research. There certainly is a safe way to fast; at the same time, ignorantly jumping into a fast is very dangerous. When executed correctly, fasting can heal many severe illnesses and diseases. I highly encourage you to research water fasting and see if it could be beneficial for you as it has been for many people throughout history.

13

FINANCES

"Wealth is the ability to fully experience life." – Henry David Thoreau

Many times throughout our lives, we uncover things that need to heal that are not biological. There can be real hardships in all categories of our personal lives, including but not limited to: relationships, careers, spirituality, sex, self-love, recreation, health, and finances. Unfortunately, the category of finances seems to dictate the wellbeing of most of those other categories. Though this book is mainly about healing from Lyme disease, I thought it was important to add a chapter on financial development in hopes that it can heal any reader's poor financial wellbeing. Most of the treatment methods discussed in this book will not be covered under medical insurance. This information will help get your finances in order so that is one less obstacle that may affect your decision-making. I am not a financial advisor or guru by any means, but I have been fortunate enough to be in a reasonably comfortable financial position through reading, listening, studying, and associating with a community of high-income financial professionals. Financial literacy has become quite a passion of mine to study and understand the tools of money and economics. I am now very passionate about helping others who are interested in putting in the effort to strengthen their financial position. If you apply some of this same information that has helped me get out from the burden of living paycheck to paycheck, you will be in a far better position to afford any of the health protocols or high-quality foods that you wish. Then you will also be in a position of strength if you would like to help others.

Have you ever asked yourself, at what point did I set the goal to get the lifestyle I have right now? Isn't it strange that people find themselves with a career that is entirely obscure from their goals or former training and education? It is as if some people just sort of end up there by happenstance. Being that I was the same way, I didn't think much of this until being introduced to the concept of intentional living. Rather than first asking, "what do I want to DO for a career..." which then defines the lifestyle you get, asking "what do I want my lifestyle to BE like..." and then finding out what action to take that will achieve that.

I learned that it has everything to do with the way you think first, and only then can you create what you have imagined in the faculty of your mind. Why wasn't I taught better thinking in school? As the old Chinese saying goes, "when the wrong man uses the right means, the right means work in the wrong way." The means I'm referring to is how we get educated. The school system in which we are indoctrinated into at such a young age. A system that does not teach us HOW to think, but where the mere memorization of facts is the determining scale of intellect. It is a shame since there are so many wonderful creative educators whose abilities are suppressed by the fiat curriculums they must teach within. It is important to recognize this is a human-made system, one in which was created with specific intent. However, most people put as much faith into it as they put into their religion, without getting results. People are working longer days, implementing double-income households, and picking up weekend gigs to maintain a similar lifestyle people used to have on one income. A system of education is absolutely needed, hence "the right *means*." But it is clearly not working in the right way.

Learning is one of life's greatest gifts. It is so important to be in a culture that is continually evolving to think at a higher frequency. But what happened to the concept of a self-directed education? Why do we feel the need to rely on the government to tell us what, or more importantly, HOW we should be learning? I want to be clear that I believe learning from others is an important part. Mentors collapse the time frames of a learning curve. Look how much debt is produced by the system that is teaching financial skills. Is it any wonder why over 50% of Americans have a negative net worth? Why do over 70% of Americans die with debt to pass to their loved ones?

The founding fathers of The United States of America all attribute their success to the copious amounts of books they studied, joining community 'Master Mind' groups (such as Ben Franklin's JUNTO), starting and failing businesses, apprenticing and mentorship, cultivating meaningful relationships, and a strong hunger for growing leadership skills and personal development. Think of the positive ripple effect that would happen in our community if that kind of education was the culture again! To quote best selling author Grant Cardone, "Although the media often discusses the disparity between the rich and the poor, they frequently fail to cover the amount of time and energy the wealthy have committed to reading, studying, and educating themselves..." This promotion of self-education does not just include financial success but education on all issues important to your life. A self-directed education is so vital to the growth of a community, to the prosperity of an economy, and the freedom of the people. In reference to the Chinese saying above, I think it's time that the right people begin using the right means so that it can work in the right way.

* * *

It may initially seem random to be discussing education, but that is where change begins. If we want better results in a specific area, we need better information to apply. Our society does not teach us financial literacy, in fact, quite the opposite. We learn how to consume our way into debt, sacrificing our futures for our immediate gratifications. We learn how to achieve a good credit score so that the banks know if you are going to be a good asset for them or not. By understanding a few primitive financial principles, you can drastically change your situation. This change will allow you to be less stressed while being able to afford the costs of healing yourself or your loved ones. As you may have guessed, your healthcare plan (if you have one) will most likely not cover many of these natural remedies. It will be entirely up to you to self-fund your healing endeavors.

It is not what you make but actually what you keep that will determine your financial success. Whether you earn $25,000 per year or $250,000 per year, it does not matter if you do not know how to manage and keep a portion of your income. I used to think that I would be in a better spot if only I could make more money. That is part of it, but I have known people with six-figure salaries that were living paycheck to paycheck and in just as much stress as someone barely working. The higher salary workers are often in more financial stress because they have much higher monthly bills, including payments to service their more substantial amounts of debt. That is usually the story behind the scenes when you hear of people you thought were doing so well completely crumble and become bankrupt, having their house and cars taken back by the banks. If you live that close to financial calamity, all it takes is a job layoff or some unexpected expense like a sick family member to topple the teetering financial tower.

The following information in this chapter includes a few fundamental principles I have been fortunate to learn, which has been a crucial aid to my healing of mind, body, and spirit. Once your finances are in good standing, you can almost put it on autopilot and use the extra time or mental capacity for more important things. It is no fun thinking about money all the time. There are so many more beautiful thoughts to be had. Money is just a magnifier; it is not good or bad. Having more money can maximize what you focus on, whether that is healing yourself, helping others, saving and investing for your children, aiding foreign countries, or simply enjoying a life of comfort. Better finances will maximize the life that you choose.

Start saving now: It does not matter how old you are or what position you are in financially. If you have any income source, begin to change your financial position by starting to save your money immediately. This principle is one of the most essential skills to develop if you want a peaceful financial situation. You may be thinking that you just can't afford to save anything because you owe it all as soon as it comes. That does not matter, skip paying the least important bill, cut back on buying lunch every day, close out your cable TV bill, make your own coffee in the morning instead of the Starbucks drive-thru. You can get creative and find ways of cutting back to pay the most important person: you, the one who is earning money. You should strive to save a minimum of ten percent of your income or more and make this a habit for the rest of your life. Eventually, your savings rate will hopefully be much higher, but if you have not been a saver until now, I would begin with ten percent and then increase from there. Any person of wealth has most likely made saving a non-negotiable habit. With this habit of saving comes opportunity. If you are a saver, you will eventually become your own bank. That will bring more options to your life.

Emergency Fund: It will take some time to sort through all the old bad spending habits, so focus on paying yourself FIRST before anyone else gets paid. Open a separate savings account and let this accumulate. This account is the beginning of what we will call an emergency fund. The goal of an emergency fund is to have around three to six months of expenses locked away in case the worst happens. That could be any financial calamity we touched on earlier. It is so important to have this fund for several reasons. First, having money in cash in the bank at the ready can dissolve certain problems quickly. If it is a health situation, you'll be able to fund that remedy for surgery or whatever it is immediately without prolonging the problem. The second reason; you will be able to quickly solve financial challenges without needing to borrow money, which can take a long time and only sink you deeper in the hole. If you total your car and need a new one, having the cash set aside can save you thousands of dollars. If you bought a $10,000.00 car in cash, that amount is your maximum cost. If you financed that same car over five years, you would end up paying almost $12,000.00. Someone with the money for that car will pay $2,000.00 less than the person that takes out a loan. This situation depicts the idea that the poor get poorer and the rich get richer.

Eliminate debt: Get out of personal debt as fast as you possibly can. If you have compound interest working against you, it will be extremely hard to get ahead. Fighting fiat inflation every year is hard enough. When you add debt interest such as school loans, mortgage, auto loans, and consumer credit cards, it makes it nearly impossible not to decline in your financial status. While continuing to save, start to pay down your highest interest rates first. Most likely, it is consumer credit cards that would be the highest; get rid of them as soon as possible. If you pay one off, use that same amount of money you paid to it every month and add that to another debt payment. This approach is called the snowball or debt-roll down method. It will be the fastest way to get out from under your debt load. You may be able also to refinance high interest rate loans for lower rates. If you do this, continue paying as much as you can per month, even if the minimum payment is less. I know paying off debt is not fun, but I can guarantee you will be decreasing your stress with every decreasing bill. This stress-reduction plays a vital role in your health. It is unlikely to heal physically while suffocating under an unbearable financial weight.

Reduce Expenses: Money saved is even more potent than the same amount of money earned as it has a double effect. It sounds obvious, but every dollar not spent is a dollar saved, whereas a dollar that needs to be earned may not be all profit to you. When you save a dollar that is already there by cutting an expense, it is 100% profit. Let's say you have a cable-TV bill of the national average amount at $85.00 per month. Now you call up your cable company and tell them you are canceling the subscription. After all the last-ditch efforts and lower priced offers to keep you around, they finally let you go. This action will not only save you $1020.00 per year of money you are already making anyway, but it also brings your expenses down by $1020.00 per year. Do you see the double effect? Sometimes, the fastest way to change your financial situation is not by launching a business or working extra hard to get a promotion at work, but to simply cut back on your unnecessary monthly expenses, which can be a lot easier than trying to get a raise!

Plug the holes in your financial boat or it will continue to sink faster than you can bail it out. If you are trading time for money, you should be cautious as you only have so much time in a day to try to catch up when you get behind. The best method for getting ahead as quickly as possible is cutting back on your expenses. I would like to share a fictional story to illuminate how cutting expenses can be much more effective than going out and trying to make more money.

The following story is from a book called *Financial Fitness* by Chris Brady and Orrin Woodward: *"John and Sally are married* *with two children. John earns $40,000 per year. With this salary alone, they were struggling each month simply to pay their bills, so Sally went out and got a job making $20,000 per year. With this 50% increase in their household income, they couldn't understand why they still seemed to struggle just as much as they did before. Follow along and see why getting that job was not very helpful.*

Based on 2013 tax rates, Sally's job created new federal and state income taxes of $4,845 and social security taxes in the amount of $1,530. She drove ten miles per day round trip, five days per week, fifty weeks per year, totaling $1,430 in commuting expenses (valued by the IRS at $.55 per mile). She spent an average of $7 per day, five days per week, fifty weeks per year on lunches totaling $1,750. She had to buy some business clothes, which needed to be dry cleaned, so that cost another $1,200 for the year. And since both John and Sally were working, neither of them wanted to make dinner when they got home, so they started eating out more often, adding another $2,000 to their food bill for the year. They needed childcare, which cost $125 per week and totaled $6,200 for the fifty weeks out of the year that Sally worked. After all of these expenditures, the couple was left with only $985 of additional income for the year!"

Looking Ahead: There are many more tools and skills in personal finance. The above are just a few important starting points that I highly recommend everyone learn to do and apply. It will radically change your finances, which can revolutionize your entire life. If you accomplish these ideas to obtain financial ease, I will encourage you to seek more financial education to take your knowledge and actions to the next level. First, you must get past survival mode of the paycheck to paycheck life. Once you are beyond the paycheck cycle, you can become debt-free and never take on any consumer debt ever again. Once your net worth is at zero with being debt-free, the clock to financial independence begins. Save as much as you can; the smaller your expenses are, the easier it is to accelerate your savings rate. Once you accumulate an excess amount of savings, you will be in a position to begin investing. That is an exciting moment; just make sure you research and learn about where you are putting your hard-earned money. There are numerous blogs, books, and podcasts from the financial independence community that will guide you to a great financial future. The goal here is not to be so focused on money that it becomes our life but rather to develop our finances and put it on autopilot to supplement the quality of life that we can all achieve. After all, that is why we are fighting through Lyme disease, right? Our health is important for our finances, and our finances are important for our health. I wish you the best of both.

14

CLOSING BLESSING

When you're lower than you've ever been, you have a chance to rise higher than you've ever risen.

I have made the statement numerous times throughout this book that I am thankful for my Lyme disease. Lyme disease has been the biggest blessing of my life. To some people, that may seem like such a strange statement, but it is true. And I don't just say that to have an attitude of gratitude, which is essential. I also do not mean blessing in a way that surrenders my autonomy to an external power. I mean, I am 100% thankful for the Lyme disease burrowing their corkscrew-shaped bodies deep into my tissue. I am glad that it destroyed me inside and out, bringing me to the brink of hopeless defeat. I feel blessed that the old me shattered into unrecognizable slivers. As a phoenix rises from the ashes, reborn into a new life, I have ascended from the puddle of despair and transformed into a new being.

Through the process of overcoming struggle came the death of untamed ego, through which has revitalized my relationships and how I perceive the world and its manifestations. I am eternally grateful for this massive awakening. It brought me out of the dark veil of ignorance and sparked the light of curiosity to question why we do anything the way that we do and ponder how it can be better. This experience has revealed the corruption, suppression, and oppression we all face within the modern world. Lyme disease has ignited a fire inside me to live prosperously and vigorously, to challenge the status quo, to break free of any self-imposed physical and mental prisons that have contained me up until now. The awakening has freed my mind, liberated my body, and revealed my spirit.

Lyme disease is just a scapegoat in this story. It has been my vehicle; however, with any extreme hardship in life, it is here to teach us, strengthen us, and evolve our spirits. Through overcoming adversity, we can become vibrant, conscious souls radiating light in a dark world. All it takes is for you to start your journey of rebirth. I am by no means more unique than the next person. If I can do this, so can you. It breaks my heart when I hear of someone who has Lyme disease that has tried everything and given up hope. I certainly was at that point for a while. I have seen Lyme's darkest nights, and I can tell you from experience that it is not impossible to one day see the light of recovery. You are stronger than you may know. If you do not think you can do this, know that is just your self-talk trying to convince you to settle. That voice is not you; it is an illusion. There will be a battle of positive and negative warring in your mind during your journey; the question is, which side will you feed? Choose positivity, choose hope, choose health. You can do this. Your body, mind, and spirit can and will get through this.

You are not alone.

We are in this together.

I believe in you.

Believe in you.

Believe.

Afterword

I truly believe everyone can heal one way or another if they put in the effort. If you had success from applying any of the information you may have learned about here in this book, it would be really great to hear from you. Please reach out to me and let me know how you are doing. I would love to hear your story.

www.AnsGibson.com

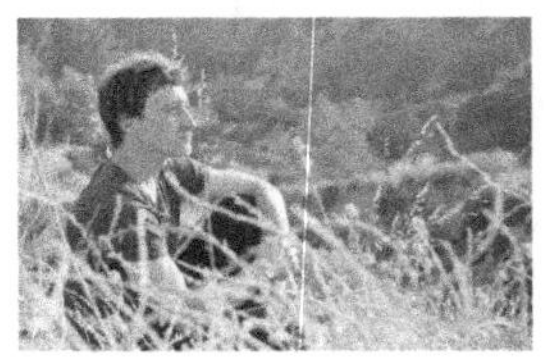

About the Author

Everybody writes their own story. However, sometimes the beginning of the story is written for us before we learn how to take back our power. Before we learn how to control our lives, the initial journey is usually a rocky, blistering road. My journey started with an intense battle of debilitating Lyme disease, which lasted nearly a decade. This struggle, which is now a tiny mirage in my rear-view mirror, has been the biggest blessing to my life. That's right; I am incredibly grateful for having and defeating Lyme disease.

The journey of overcoming the illness has completely reshaped my thinking and what I have learned has revolutionized my lifestyle. There I was, at the age of 28 years old, completely reborn! At that time, I began to wonder, how could I give back this amazing gift? How can I help other suffering souls in this world? I believe in the droplets-in-a-bucket mindset; we each can do one small thing in our lives to purify our droplets and the few droplets around us until eventually, the whole bucket is pure. What I feel called to do is promote and encourage this information to those who are open to change and begin their journey toward healing themselves. My focus is on the positivity and hope needed to begin a healing journey and to hopefully inspire the community to promote this critical information in the same magical, loving way that it changed my life. Love and best wishes throughout your Lyme disease recovery. - Ans Gibson, Author, and Founder of TrueVeganLove.com.